MW01382157

An Atlas of
AMPLITUDE-INTEGRATED EEGs IN THE NEWBORN

An Atlas of
AMPLITUDE-INTEGRATED EEGs IN THE NEWBORN

Lena Hellström-Westas

Department of Pediatrics, University Hospital

Lund, Sweden

Linda S. de Vries

Department of Neonatology, Wilhelmina Children's Hospital

Utrecht, The Netherlands

Ingmar Rosén

Department of Clinical Neurophysiology, University Hospital

Lund, Sweden

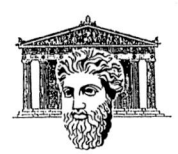

The Parthenon Publishing Group

International Publishers in Medicine, Science & Technology

A CRC PRESS COMPANY

BOCA RATON   LONDON   NEW YORK   WASHINGTON, D.C.

Published in the USA by
The Parthenon Publishing Group
345 Park Avenue South
10th Floor
New York, NY 10010
USA

Published in the UK and Europe by
The Parthenon Publishing Group
23–25 Blades Court
Deodar Road
London SW15 2NU
UK

Library of Congress Cataloging-in-Publication Data

Hellström-Westas, L. (Lena)
    An atlas of amplitude-integrated EEGs in the newborn / L. Hellström-Westas, L. de
Vries and I. Rosen.
      p. ; cm. -- (The encyclopedia of visual medicine series)
    Includes bibliographical references and index.
    ISBN 1-84214-111-2 (alk. paper)
      1. Infants (Newborn)--Abnormalities--Diagnosis--Atlases. 2.
Electroencephalography--Atlases. 3. Brain--Diseases--Diagnosis--Atlases. I. De Vries,
L. S. II. Rosen, I. (Ingmar) III. Title. IV. Series.
      [DNLM: 1. Brain--Infant, Newborn--Atlases. 2. Brain Diseases--diagnosis--Infant,
Newborn--Atlases. 3. Electroencephalography--Infant, Newborn--Atlases. WS 17 H477a 2002]
    RJ255 .H456 2002
    618.62'01-dc21   2002030356

British Library Cataloguing in Publication Data

Hellström-Westas, L.
    An atlas of amplitude-integrated EEGs in the newborn. -
    (The encyclopedia of visual medicine series)
    1. Infants (Newborn) - Diseases - Diagnosis
    2. Electroencephalography
    I. Title II. De Vries, L. S. III. Rosen, I.
    618.9'28047547

ISBN 1-84214-111-2

First published in 2003

Composition by The Parthenon Publishing Group
Additional reproduction by Graphic Reproductions, UK
Printed and bound by T. G. Hostench S.A., Spain

Contents

Abbreviations

aEEG	amplitude-integrated EEG
CFAM	Cerebral Function Analysing Monitor
CFM	Cerebral Function Monitor
CNV	Continuous normal voltage aEEG in full-term infant
CSA	Compressed spectral array
CTG	Cardiotocography
DNV	Discontinuous normal voltage aEEG in full-term infant
ECG	Electrocardiography
ECMO	Extracorporeal membrane oxygenation
EEG	Electroencephalography
EP	Evoked potential
FFT	Fast Fourier Transformation
HIE	Hypoxic–ischemic encephalopathy
GMH–IVH	Germinal matrix–intraventricular hemorrhage
ICH	Intracranial hemorrhage
ICU	Intensive care unit
Lido	Lidocaine
Mida	Midazolam
MRI	Magnetic resonance imaging
NICU	Neonatal intensive care unit
PDA	Persistent ductus arteriosus
Phenob	Phenobarbitone
Phen	Phenytoin
PROM	Premature rupture of membranes
PVL	Periventricular leukomalacia
RDS	Respiratory distress syndrome
REM	Rapid eye movement
SE	Spectral edge
SEP	Somatosensory evoked potential
TTTS	Twin–twin transfusion syndrome
VEP	Visual evoked potential

Preface

As we have gained experience with the cerebral function monitor (CFM) over the years, it has given us so much valuable clinical information about our patients that we are convinced that it should be available for all newborn intensive care patients.

The technique was introduced in Lund in 1978 after Ingmar Rosén had visited Pamela Prior in London to discuss a method for experimental EEG monitoring. At that time there were several publications on the use of the CFM in adults. Ingmar Rosén, together with Nils Svenningsen, felt that there was a need for more intensive monitoring of brain function in their very vulnerable newborn babies and they were encouraged to try using the monitor. A few years later Lena Hellström-Westas, with the assistance of Ingmar Rosén and Nils Svenningsen, started to evaluate the method in the neonatal intensive care unit (NICU). Linda de Vries visited Lund in 1992 to learn to use the CFM and to interpret the recordings. At that time there were four CFM machines in Lund. Within a few years Utrecht had six machines.

At that stage we had no plans to write an atlas of CFM monitoring together. However, with the increasing use of the CFM all over the world, particularly for the prognosis of asphyxia in the term infant and for selection for intervention studies on, for example, hypothermia for perinatal asphyxia, it has become clear that there is a need for a reference atlas. We also wanted to have an opportunity to give examples of the use of the CFM in other clinical situations.

We planned to write the *Atlas of Amplitude-Integrated EEGs in the Newborn* together with Nils Svenningsen. Sadly, he died suddenly before we could start the work. He was and is a great inspiration to us and we are dedicating this Atlas to his memory.

We are grateful to the many people who have worked on developing and promoting the use of the CFM. First, we want to thank Pamela Prior for introducing the method to us and for generously sharing her experience of the CFM with us. We also want to thank Douglas Maynard for his discussions on CFM development and on the Cerebral Function Analysing Monitor (CFAM). We thank Marianne Thoresen who, together with Douglas Maynard, contributed a nice CFAM example. We are also grateful for stimulating CFM discussions with Klara Thiringer, Eva Thornberg, Gorm Greisen and Denis Azzopardi and for all the input we have received from CFM sessions at the European Neonatal Brain Club. In order to stress the utility of a method rather than a commercially available machine, we have applied Gorm Greisen's term 'amplitude-integrated EEG' (aEEG) throughout the Atlas.

Introducing the CFM into our NICUs was easy and all the neonatologists quickly learned to interpret the traces. We would like to thank Floris Groenendaal, Paula Eken, Karin Rademaker, Kristina Thorngren-Jerneck, Helena Klette and, especially, Mona Toet all of whom have contributed to publications that are quoted in the Atlas. We are also grateful to Kees van Huffelen who helped to compare the CFM and the standard EEG. We are happy for and much appreciate all technical assistance and support that we received from May Vitestam, Elin Persson, Paul Mikkelsen and Lars-Johan Ahnlide. Much of this work could not have been done without the enthusiastic support of all the nurses in our units who quickly learned how to attach the monitor to a baby, obtain a good recording and to appreciate the significance of the traces. Thanks go especially to Marianne Buikema and Joke Zoet who were involved in producing a wonderful teaching CD Rom.

Finally, we hope that many babies will benefit from this Atlas and that the reader will find it a practical reference, a good learning experience and have as much fun going through it as we had putting it together.

Lena Hellström-Westas
Linda S. de Vries
Ingmar Rosén

Foreword

Every neonatologist has experienced the feeling of success when overcoming death by skilful use of mechanical ventilation, guided by blood gas measurements and pulse oximetry monitoring. Many neonatologists have felt the disappointment when this feeling of success is gradually replaced by sadness when a surviving child develops ever more evident signs of severe brain injury. Therefore, neonatologists are concerned about the well-being of the brain of their patients under intensive care, because brain injury is an ever-present threat to newborn patients.

There is a disproportion between the wealth of methods for monitoring respiratory function, and the paucity of methods for monitoring brain function. Respiration and gas exchange are targets for intervention, and oxygenation and acid–base balance are prerequisites for normal brain function. If we had a respirator for the brain, with which we could manage electroencephalography (EEG), there can be no doubt that the amplitude-integrated EEG (aEEG) would already be a well-served tool in neonatology. After all, it was invented 40 years ago. You do a favor to the brain by being careful with the management of respiration, but you do it blind. If you are really concerned, there is no substitute for trying to find out.

In a term baby under intensive care because of critical respiratory failure, who has been exposed to one or more episodes of hypoxia–ischemia, a normal trace of aEEG is a simple and efficient means of documenting whether it is worthwhile carrying on. There is probably no other way to obtain this information.

Clearly, once you start monitoring aEEGs you will face problems that you did not have before. What do you do about electrical seizures without clinical signs? How do you inform the parents of a very preterm baby with persistently discontinuous activity? How can you be sure that what you see on the paper trace is really EEG, and not just noise and artefacts?

This book comes in as a first: brief, practical and useful to the busy neonatologist. The authors have used aEEG for years in research. In Lund, the first use of this technology grew from the fruitful collaboration of a careful neonatologist, the late Nils Svenningsen, and a neurophysiologist, Ingmar Rosén, who was prepared to give up the methodological stringency of multi-lead EEG to get functional monitoring of the brain into around-the-clock neonatal practice. Lena Hellström-Westas carried out most of the consolidating work; Linda deVries showed that the technology could be transferred without losing its sharpness. aEEG is part of daily practice in Lund and Utrecht. The book is written out of this experience.

Gorm Greisen
Professor of Paediatrics
Juliane Marie Centre
Rigshospitalet, Copenhagen, Denmark

1

Methodology

Continuous electroencephalography (EEG) monitoring is a relatively new modality in intensive care in general as well as in neonatal intensive care. Whereas a number of physiological parameters such as electrocardiography (ECG), heart rate, oxygen saturation, blood pressure and temperature have long since been integrated into intensive care unit (ICU) monitoring systems, monitoring of EEGs, directly reflecting the functional state of the brain, has been used more rarely. There are probably a number of reasons for this:

(1) The EEG signal is of low amplitude and often contaminated by artefacts of biological and non-biological origin. Interpretation of the EEG requires long and extensive experience with due consideration given to a number of factors such as level of wakefulness and medication given, and, in neonatal patients, to gestational age and activity state.

(2) It is almost impossible for the attending clinician or nurse to extract useful trends in the development of the functional state of the brain during intensive care by inspecting the ongoing EEG activity only.

(3) Even for the professional EEG interpreter it is very difficult to discern trends of EEG development during hours and days of intensive care by repeated inspection of the ongoing raw EEG signal displayed on a time-scale, which is usually in the order of 10–20 s per page.

(4) Furthermore, the intensive care situation does not permit maintenance of impedance and position of multiple EEG recording electrodes on the scalp for any length of time exceeding a few hours.

These considerations have inspired a number of developments in monitoring devices, which provide simplified time-compressed displays of EEGs during intensive care. The two main physical features of the EEG signal that are targeted, are variations in the amplitude (amplitude-integrated EEG (aEEG)) and frequency content (compressed spectral arrays (CSA), spectral edge).

The EEG is a spatiotemporal average of synchronous post-synaptic potentials in cortical pyramidal cells oriented in parallel. Synchronous neuronal activity arises by various mechanisms. Individual thalamocortical relay cells, cells in the thalamic reticular nucleus and cortical pyramidal cells each have endogenous recurrent action potential firing properties[1]. The activity within groups of thalamocortical neurones is synchronized by recurrent connections between thalamocortical relay cells and the surrounding reticular thalamic nucleus and between the thalamus and cortex. During arousal, cholinergic (and noradrenergic) afferents from the brainstem exert an excitatory depolarizing effect on thalamocortical and cortical cells and inhibit the reticular thalamic cells. The net result of arousal is a reduction of synchronous activity and an increase of asynchronous high-frequency activity as is illustrated in Figure 1.1, recorded from an awake full-term newborn infant at rest and during verbal stimulation.

Maynard originally constructed the cerebral function monitor (CFM) in the late 1960s in response to need in intensive care for continuous EEG monitoring. Its clinical applications, mainly in adult patients during anesthesia and in intensive care, e.g. after cardiac arrest, during status epilepticus and after heart surgery, were developed by Prior[2–4]. Critikon (Florida, USA) and Lectromed (Letchworth, UK) produced versions of the CFM. The technique and major clinical applications of the CFM are summarized in the book *Monitoring Cerebral Function: Long Term Monitoring of EEG and Evoked Potentials* by P.F. Prior and D.E. Maynard, published by Elsevier, Amsterdam, 1986, to which the reader is referred for details[5]. In the present Atlas we have used the term aEEG to denote a method for electrocortical monitoring rather than a specific machine. However, most examples are from cerebral function monitors.

The EEG signal for the aEEG is recorded from one channel (optional two channels) with two symmetrical parietal electrodes, or bilateral fronto-parietal electrodes. The signal is amplified and passed through an asymmetrical band-pass filter which strongly attenuates activity below 2 Hz and above 15 Hz in order to minimize artefacts from, for example, sweating and muscle activity, ECG and electrical interference (Figure 1.2). With the high-pass filter set at 2 Hz a significant part of the low-frequency components of the neonatal EEG signal is attenuated.

Between 2 and 15 Hz the filter shape compensates for the fact that the electrical energy of the non-rhythmic components of the EEG signal tends to decrease with increase of frequency (approximately 12 dB/decade)[3]. The EEG processing includes semilogarithmic amplitude compression, rectifying, smoothing with a time constant of 0.5 s and time compression (Figure 1.2).

The band width in the output reflects variations in minimum and maximum EEG amplitude (Figure 1.3). The semilogarithmic output enhances changes in background activity of very low (< 5 μV) amplitudes. The signal is written out on slow speed, 6 cm/h or 30 cm/h in the CFM 4640 and from 1 mm/min to 100 mm/s in the CFM Multitrace 2. The paper speed in the CFM examples in this Atlas is 6 cm/h unless stated otherwise.

The input impedance is recorded simultaneously on a second channel. Scalp muscle activity may be detected by its interference with the impedance detector. Overload of the recording system either by a direct current (DC) offset or by excessive alternate current (AC) potentials (> 800 μV peak to peak) will cut out both recorder channels and an overload-indicator lamp is lit. Extracerebral sources of signals below this level and falling within the frequency window of the recorder will add to the aEEG signal displayed with a risk of misinterpretation as a result.

A critical change of brain perfusion or metabolism markedly affects the amplitude and power of the EEG signal, whereas more gradual and moderate changes primarily affect the frequency content of the EEG. This is illustrated in Figure 1.4 with a comparison of the CFM–aEEG trace with a raw EEG recorded before, during, and at restitution after severe experimental hypoglycemia in rat[6]. At the onset of hypoglycemia (trace 2), the amplitude of the EEG signal increases with an increase particularly of the low-frequency EEG components. This causes a moderate increase of the CFM signal. More severe hypoglycemia results in a discontinuous or burst-suppression pattern (trace 3) reflecting a disconnection of the function of the thalamocortical neuronal circuitry. In the CFM, the minimum level of the trace approaches the zero line, whereas the maximum level is maintained. A period of complete electrocerebral inactivity (trace 4) ensues. The recovery of the EEG after glucose infusion is initiated by a brief period of seizure activity with repeated sharp waves (trace 5). In the CFM trace, this is seen as an abrupt increase from the zero line. During the subsequent recovery, the frequency content of the EEG changes from predominantly low frequency (trace 6) to mixed frequencies (trace 7) accompanied by only minor changes in the CFM trace.

The amplitude of the EEG, and therefore of the aEEG signal, is dependent on the positioning of the recording electrodes at the scalp and on the inter-electrode distance. The recommended positions of the two recording electrodes over the mid-parietal area on each side are shown in Figure 1.5. The electrodes shown are thin subdermal needles, which in our experience produce a stable and artefact-free recording for hours and even days. The very thin needle electrodes produce no, or very little, discomfort. Any conventional EEG electrodes or disposable EEG electrodes can be used as alternatives.

Decreasing the interelectrode distance will cause a decrease in the EEG signal as illustrated in Figure 1.6a. Due to the logarithmic or semilogarithmic display of the aEEG and the CFM, moderate changes in the amplitude of continuous EEG activity will not show up clearly. With alternative positions of recording electrodes, and alternative interelectrode distances, different amplitude levels of the aEEG–CFM trace will be attained (Figure 1.6b). Increased amounts of extracranial fluid between electrodes, i.e. cephalic hematomas, would decrease the recorded EEG signal due to shunting of the electric current (see Figure 3.4 in Chapter 3). aEEG monitoring from one biparietal channel does not provide any information about hemispheric asymmetries and independent recording from one channel on each side may be of clinical significance (see Figures 3.7, 3.8, 6.6 and 7.17 in later chapters), unless the aEEG monitoring is complemented with conventional EEG recording from multiple electrodes. For early recognition of focal pathological abnormalities and asymmetries in the EEG, we recommend full routine EEG at an early stage of care.

Spectral analysis of the frequency content of the EEG signal using Fast Fourier Transformation (FFT) has for a long time been the predominant electrophysiological method for monitoring anesthesia. Trend analysis is made possible by vertical stacking of sequential spectra forming a CSA. CSA of EEG is often included as a module in general commercial ICU monitoring systems. It has been used for the monitoring of clinical coma in adult patients[7]. The method has also been used in neonatal monitoring of seizures[8] and effects of treatment[9]. Seizures are recognized as episodes of increased power output (Figure 1.7c). Transient changes in the EEG signals may be squeezed into the spectral line and may not be recognizable as distinct events. A few comparative studies with aEEG methods have been reported[10–14]. No advantage was found for the Cerebro Trac technique, using FFT and spectral-edge analysis, over CFM for neonatal cerebral surveillance[15]. On the other hand, recent experimental and clinical studies

indicate that CSA and spectral-edge frequency may predict development of white matter injury in preterm infants[16].

The Cerebral Function Analysing Monitor (CFAM) is a further development of the CFM[5,17]. In addition to aEEG monitoring from two or four (CFAM3™, RDM Consultants) channels using a similar algorithm as CFM, a frequency analysis is performed and presented as percentage activity within each of the classic frequency bands and a suppression band, i.e. the percentage time the weighted EEG is below a preset value (Figure 1.8). Its use in neonatal monitoring[18] and in pediatric intensive care[19] has been documented.

Ideally, the aEEG or CSA transformation of the EEG signal used in a time-compressed mode for trend analysis at the cot-side should be stored together with the raw EEG signal. This makes it possible to identify and trace artefacts and to identify, more specifically, the character of seizure patterns and other EEG features such as interictal or short-duration seizure discharges. The CFAM technique allows for intermittent displays of the raw EEG. A system has been described for *post hoc* analysis of two channels of EEG recorded with the Medilog recorder[20]. Although useful for quantitative studies the system does not provide online cot-side trend data. Recently, digital EEG monitoring systems have been developed which allow the raw EEG to be displayed and stored continuously with online trend analysis of the aEEG (Figure 1.7a and b) as well as the CSA (reference 21 and unpublished data, Hellström-Westas and colleagues; Figure 1.9).

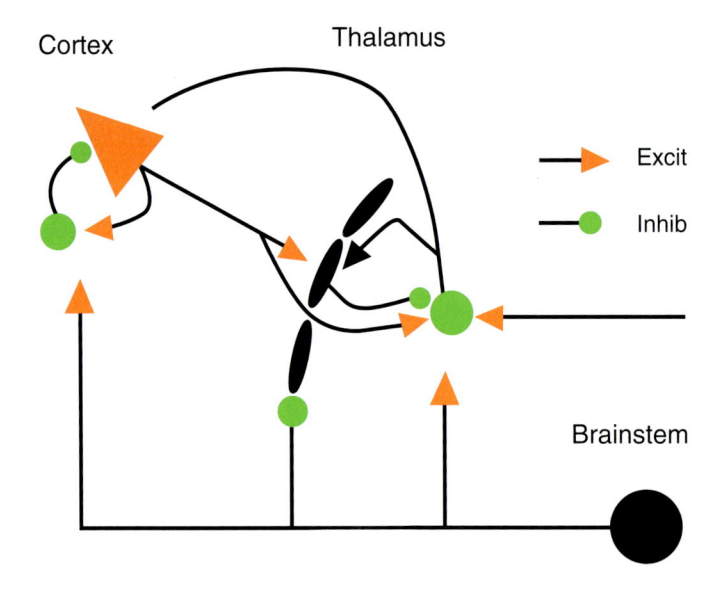

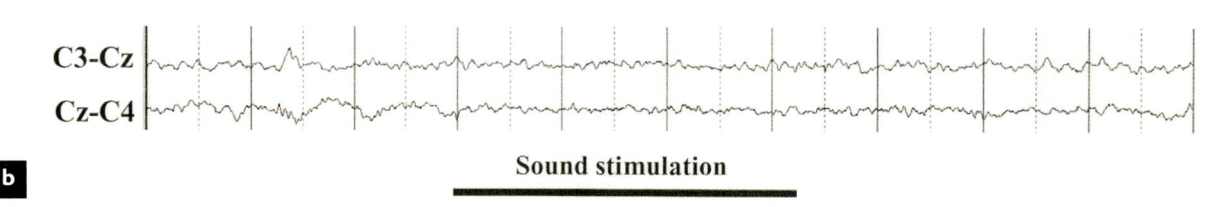

Figure 1.1 (a) A schematic diagram of the main thalamocortical neuronal circuits that are responsible for EEG rhythms. For further details, see text. (b) EEG recording from an awake term infant at rest and during auditory stimulation. Note the reduction of low-frequency EEG components at arousal

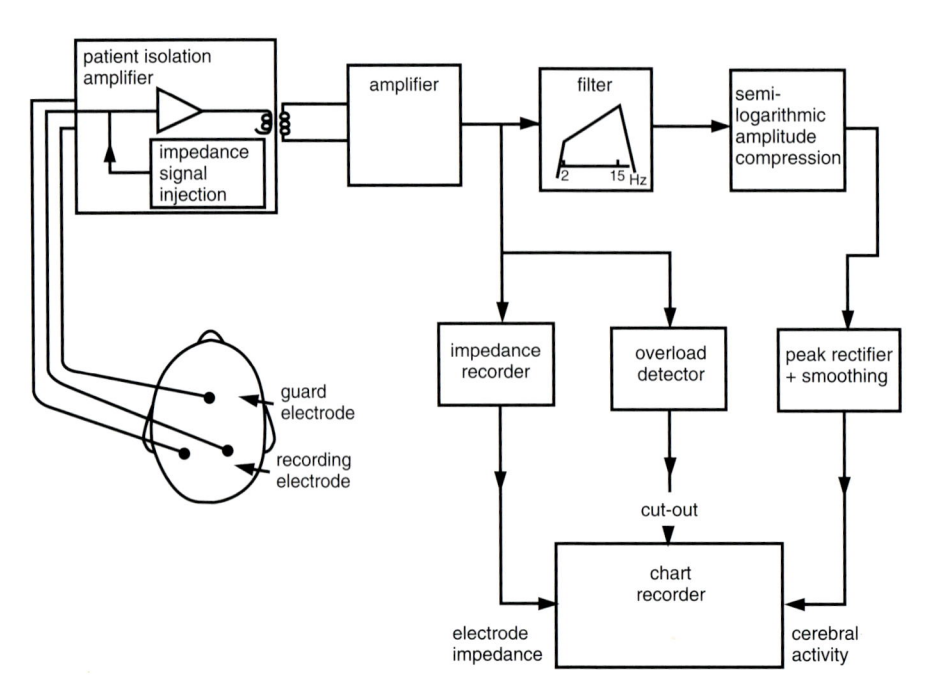

Figure 1.2 Block diagram showing signal pathways in the CFM (Type 4640). For details, see text. Reproduced from reference 5 with kind permission of the authors

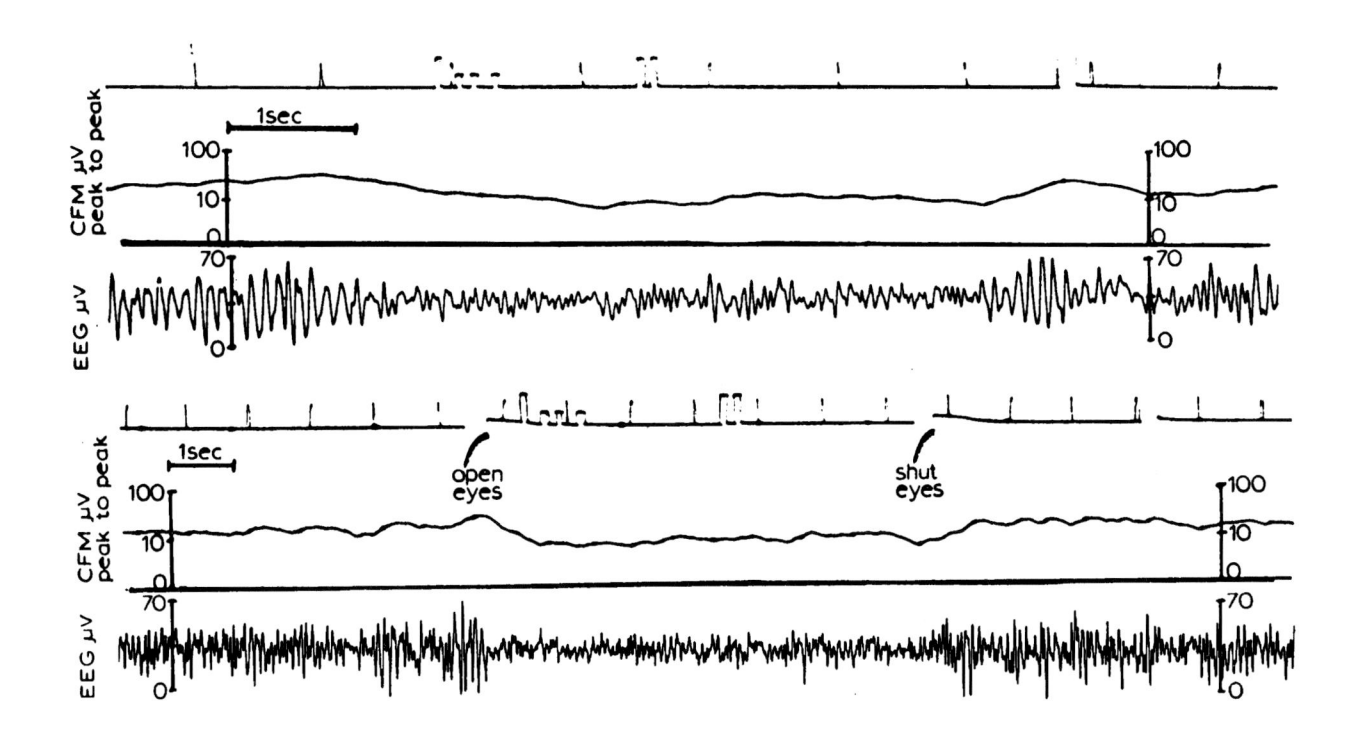

Figure 1.3 Illustration showing how the CFM output follows the amplitude fluctuations of the EEG from an awake adult subject. The CFM output has been plotted at the same speed as the EEG instead of at the usual 6 or 30 cm/h. Reproduced from reference 5 by kind permission of the authors

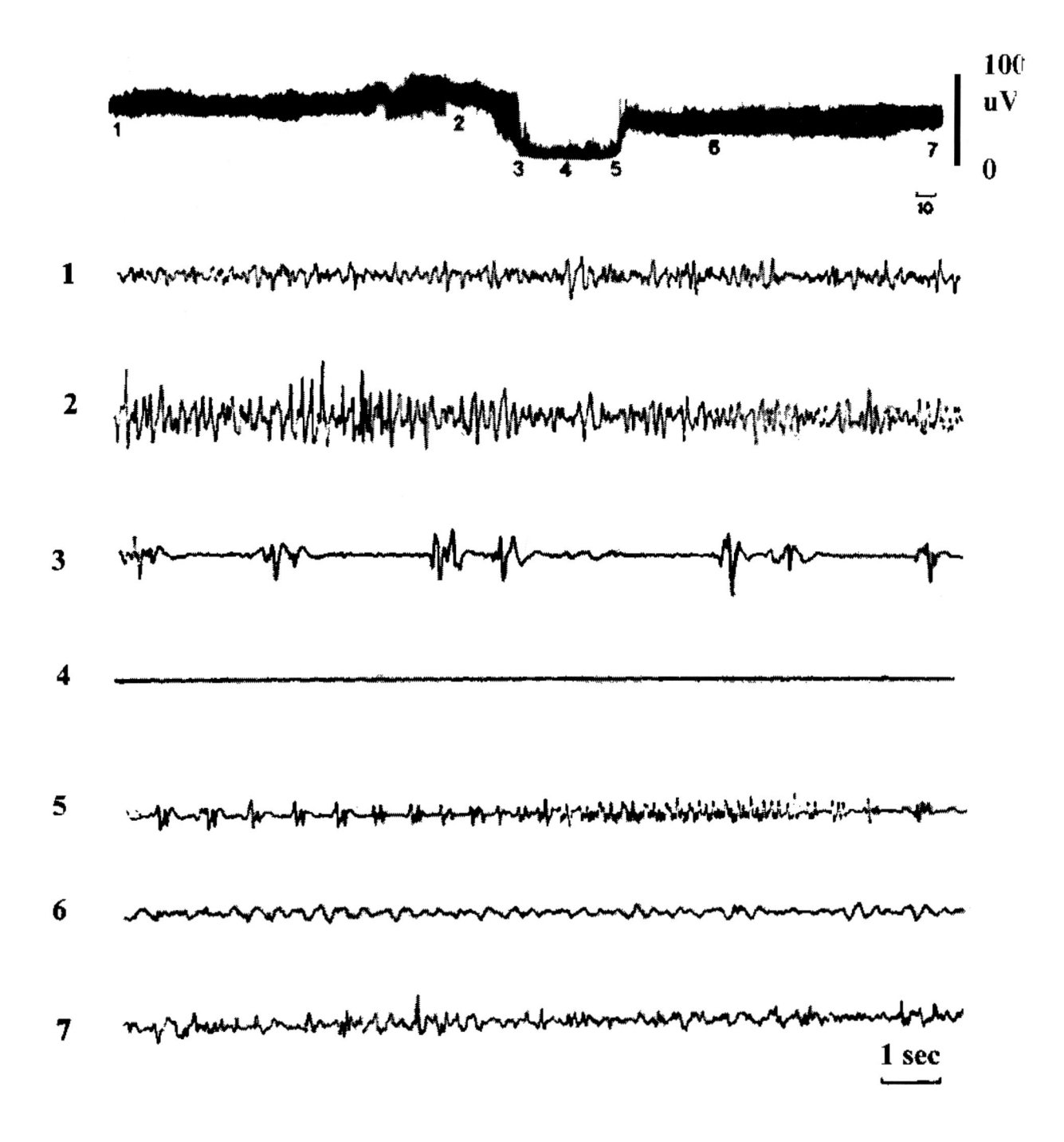

Figure 1.4   Comparison of a continuous CFM record and samples of EEG recorded from a rat before, during and after a period of severe hypoglycemia induced by insulin given intraperitoneally. The blood glucose level was restored by intravenous glucose. For further details, see text. Reproduced from reference 6 with permission

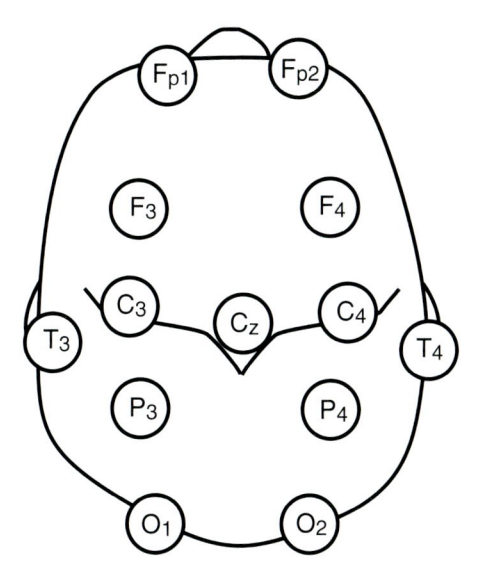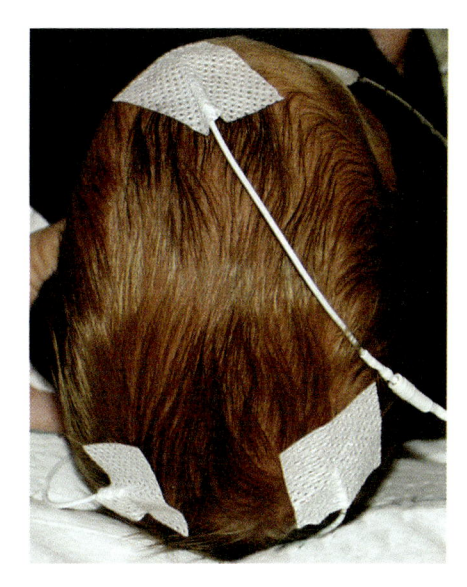

Figure 1.5 The biparietal recording electrodes P3 and P4, according to the international 10–20 system[22,23], are the recommended positions for single-channel CFM recording. Specific measurements from bony landmarks are used to determine the placement of electrodes and distances are subdivided in 10 or 20% intervals. The vertex is defined as the intersection of the line joining the top of the nose (nasion) to the external occipital protuberance (inion), and the line joining the external auditory meati. In adults, P3 and P4 are approximately 5 cm posterior to the vertex and about 8 cm apart. In a full-term neonatal infant the approximate corresponding figures are 3 and 6 cm, respectively. The neutral electrode reduces the amount of electrical interference and is positioned to the anterior in the midline.

The reason for selecting a biparietal recording for one-channel aEEG monitoring is that the underlying cerebral cortex is in the boundary zone of blood perfusion from the posterior, middle and cerebral arteries and sensitive to ischemia caused by a systemic fall in blood pressure. This location is also least likely to be affected by scalp muscle activity, and is also least affected by eye-movement artefacts

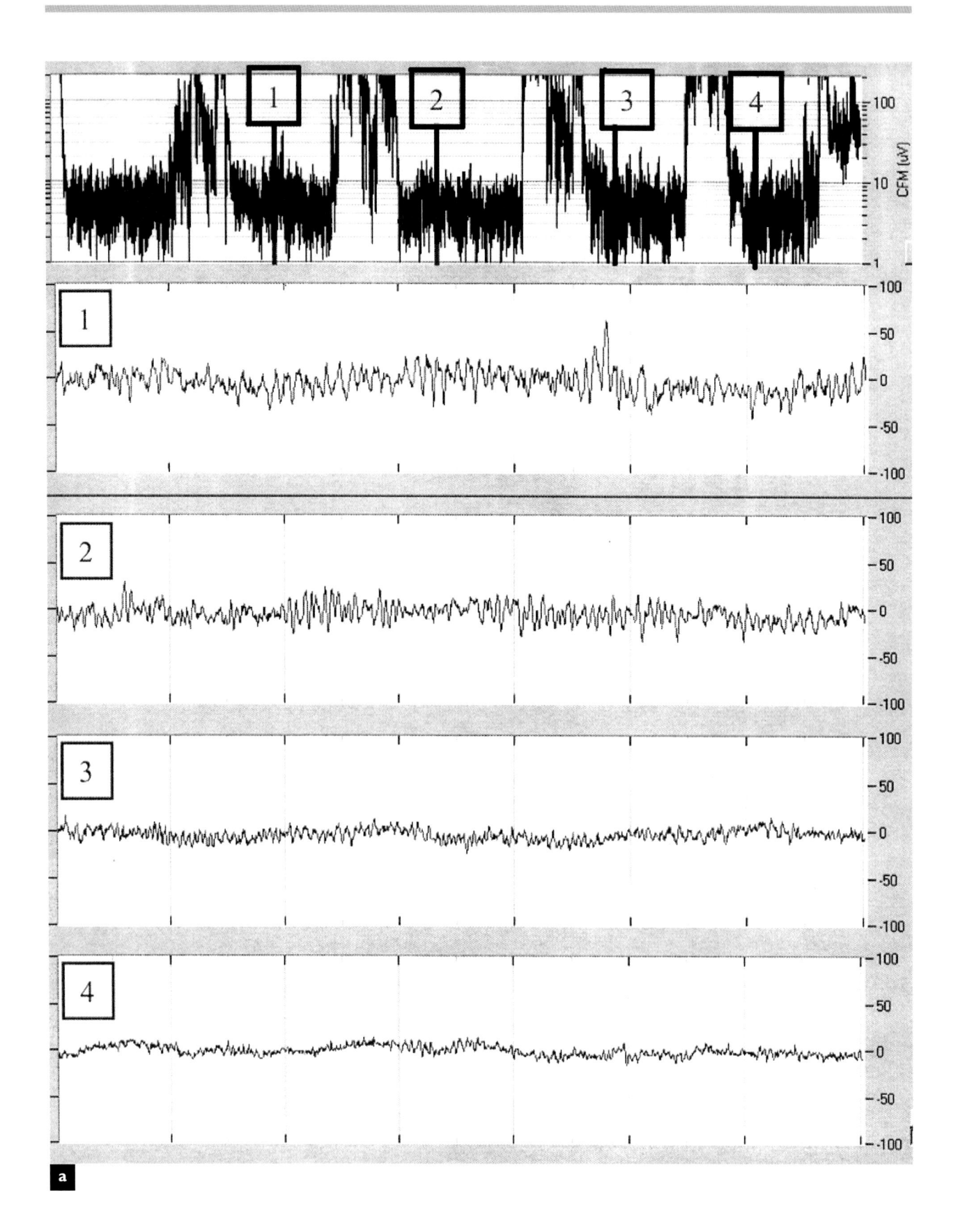

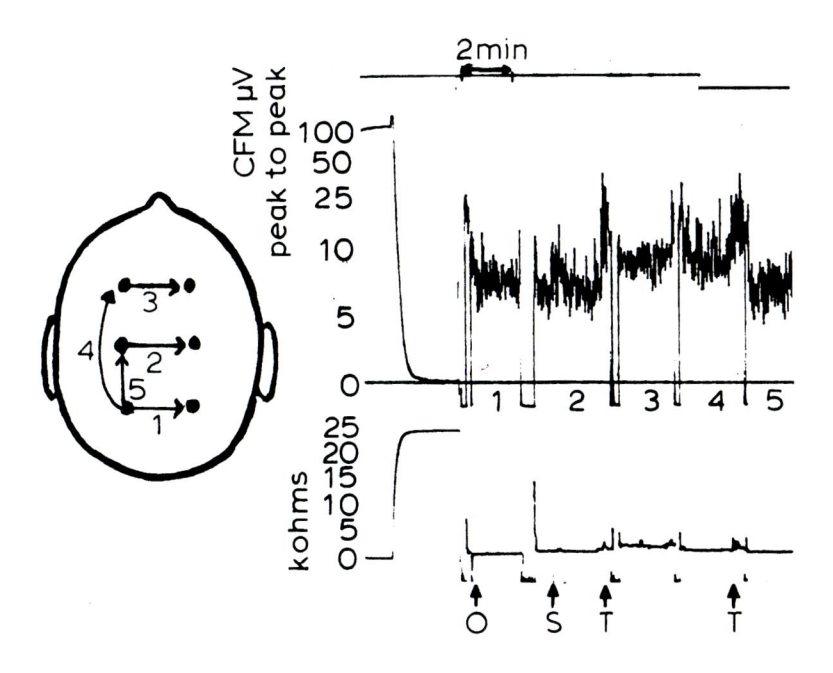

Figure 1.6 *opposite and above* (a) Sequential recording of an amplitude-integrated EEG (logarithmic display) and EEG signal with decreasing interelectrode recording distance. 1, P7–P8; 2, P5–P6; 3, P3–P4; 4, P1–P2, according to the modified 10–20 system. The progressive decrease of the EEG amplitude is clearly visible in the EEG records but is much less clear in the aEEG traces, due to the logarithmic display. Courtesy of L.J. Ahnlide.

(b) Sequential CFM recordings from five electrode derivations, demonstrating effects of electrode positions on the amplitude of the CFM trace. Interelectrode distances are 12 cm (1), 15 cm (2), 12 cm (3), 12 cm (4) and 7.5 cm (5). The annotations indicate: O, eyes open; S, eyes shut; T, talking. Samples 3 and 4 are contaminated by considerable eye-movement artefact. Scalp muscle potentials and electrode-movement artefact (on the lower electrode impedance trace) coincide with eye and facial movement; derivations 1 and 5 are the most satisfactory. Reproduced from reference 5 by kind permission of the authors

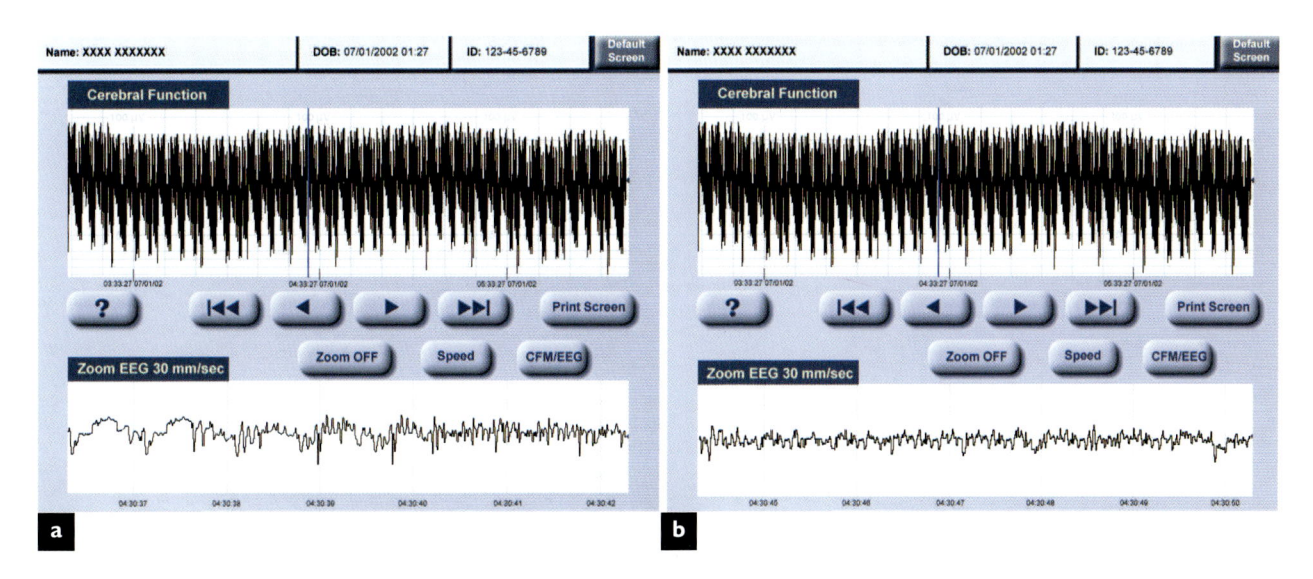

Figure 1.7 Example of simultaneous display of digital CFM and raw EEG from the recent update to the CFM 4640, the CFM 6000 (Olympic Medical). The upper display shows a characteristic CFM pattern of status epilepticus. The lower, raw-EEG signal shows (a) onset of, and (b) continuation of seizure activity. The simultaneous EEG is taken at the points indicated by the markers on the CFM trace

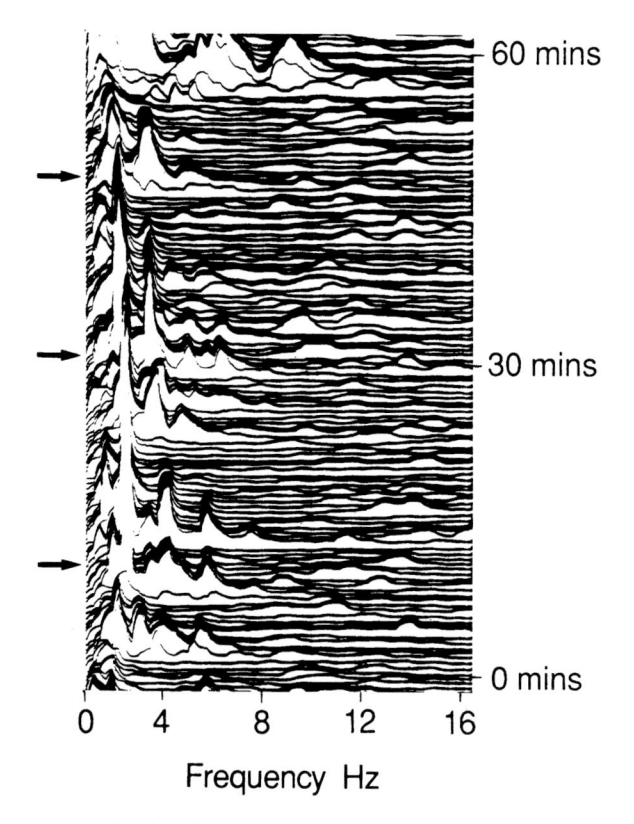

c

Figure 1.7 continued   (c) CSA–EEG display from an infant, showing continuing, intermittent, subclinical seizure activity, as indicated by the arrows. Reproduced from reference 9 with permission

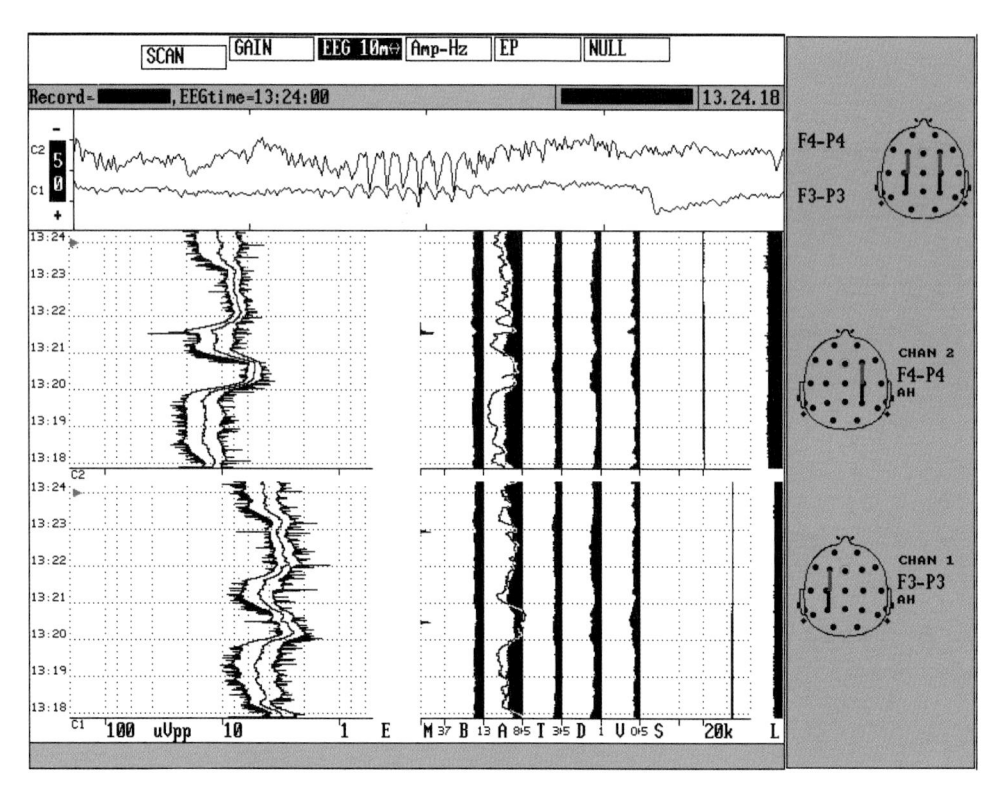

a

Figure 1.8   (a) CFAM recording (courtesy of M. Thoresen and D. Maynard) of a growth-restricted infant of 27 weeks' gestation. The infant had bronchopulmonary dysplasia, which was treated with systemic corticosteroids, and moderate hypertension. At 3 weeks of age the infant suddenly collapsed and developed rhythmic right-sided seizures

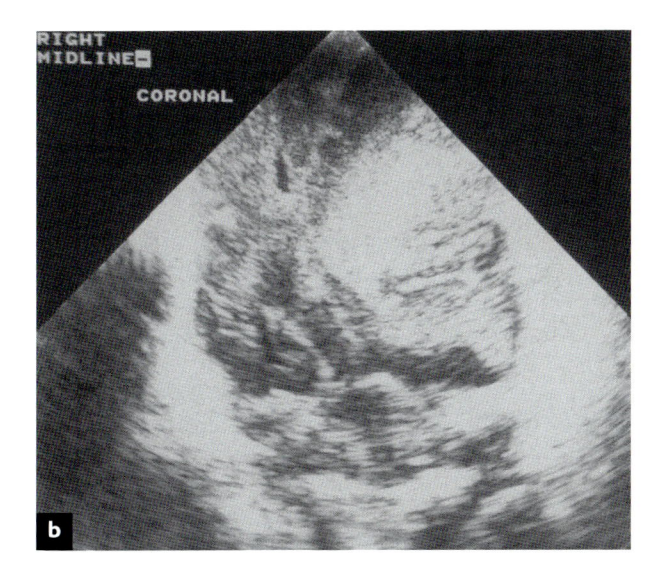 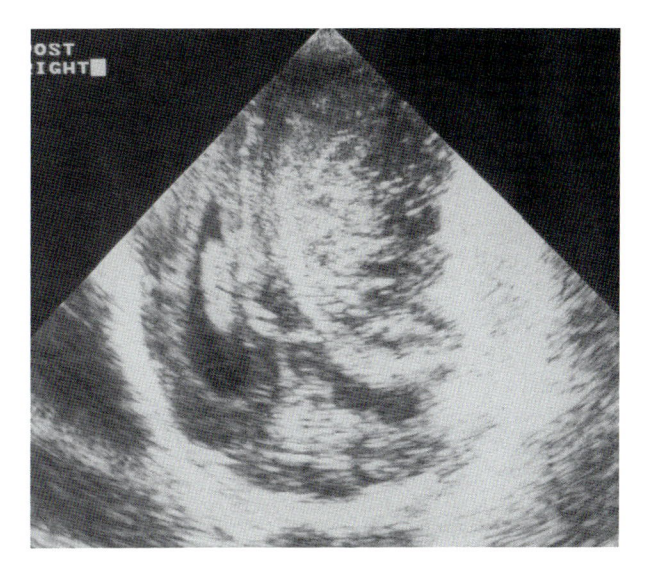

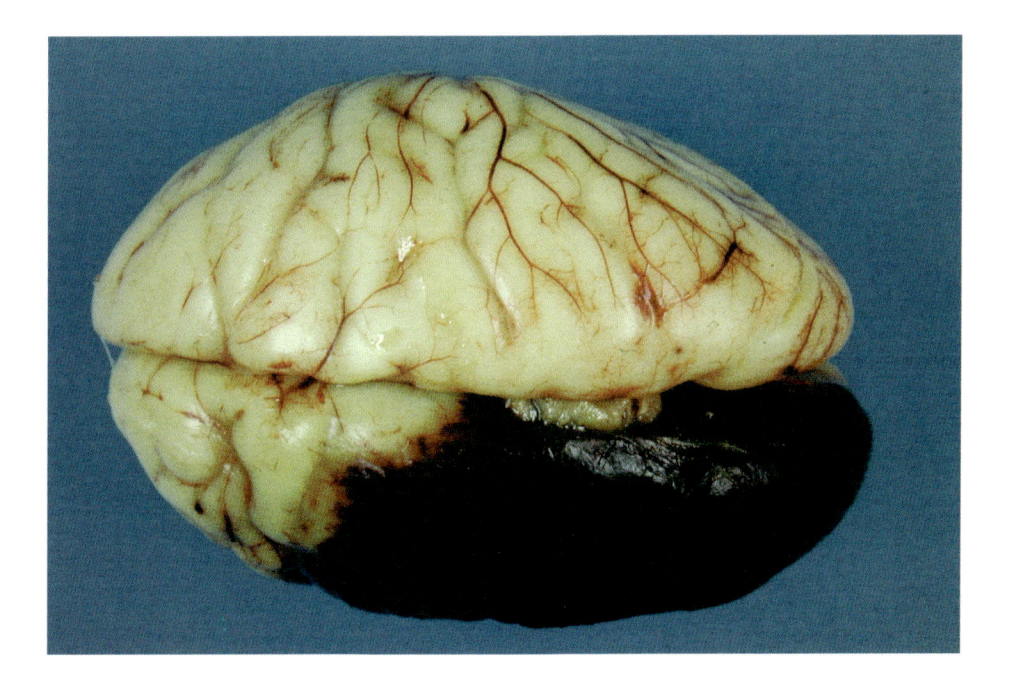

Figure 1.8 continued   (b) A cranial ultrasound (coronal midline and posterior images) demonstrated a large unilateral hemorrhage on the left side with midline shift to the right. Intensive care treatment was withdrawn.

(c) A unilateral subpial hemorrhage with parenchymal extension was confirmed at autopsy.

The bilateral CFAM3 tracing shows an asymmetrical recording with lower amplitude on the affected left side. Periods of higher amplitude in the trend monitor corresponded to times during which the comb-like EEG waves seen above were occurring. There was a 50-Hz interference, particularly on the right; this was filtered from the EEG and is outside the range of frequencies used for amplitude-frequency analysis

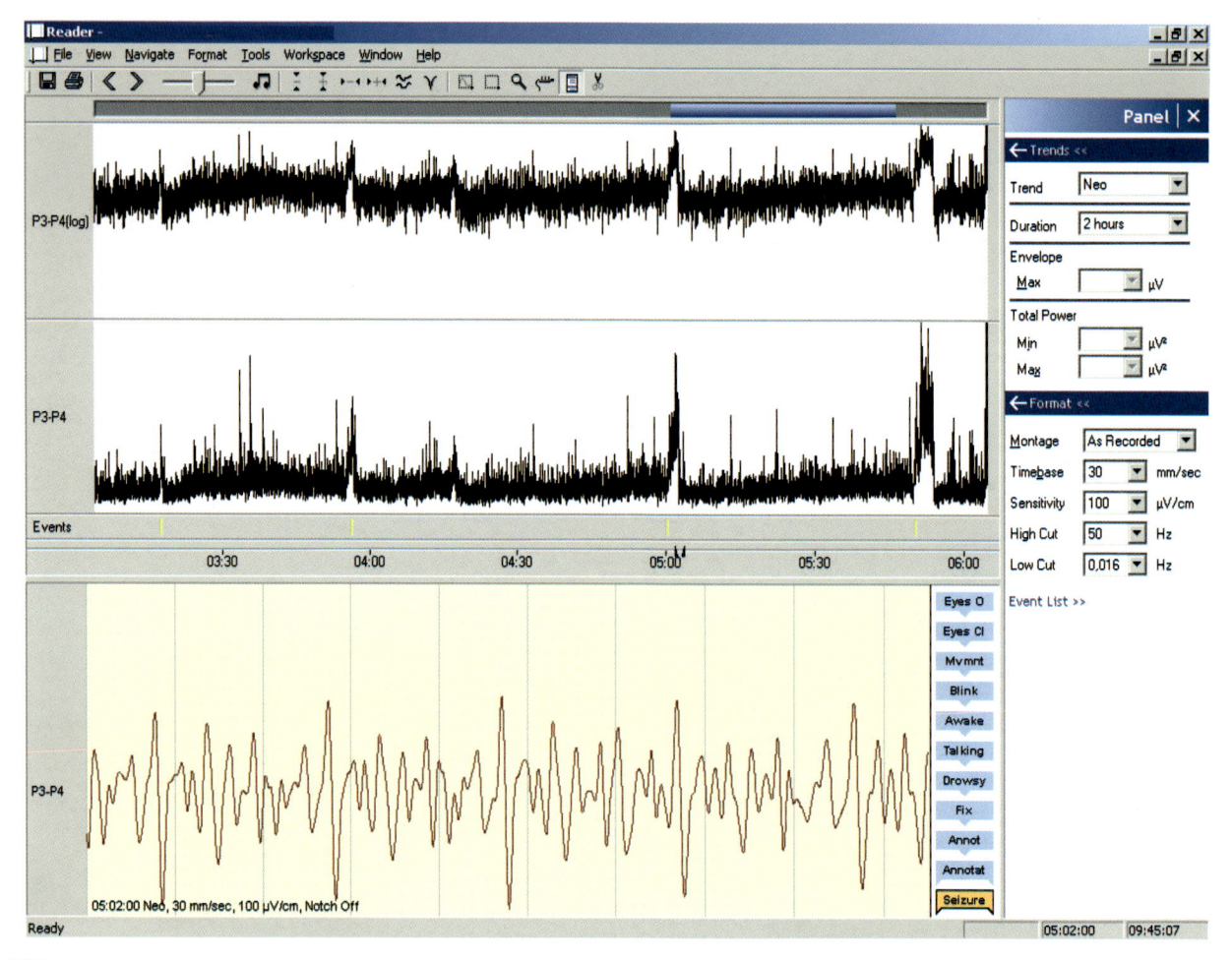

a

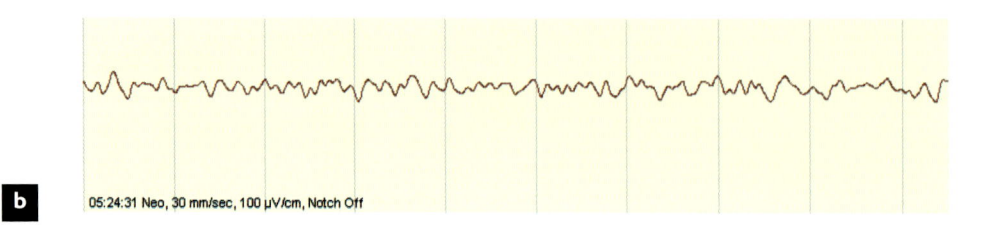

b
05:24:31 Neo, 30 mm/sec, 100 µV/cm, Notch Off

Figure 1.9 (a) Screen image of the new Nervus™ monitor (Taugagreining hf, Reykjavik, Iceland) showing an infant with continuous electrocortical background pattern with five seizures, shown as transient increases in the background activity. The raw EEG is displayed below the two trend recordings, both showing the same rectified, time-compressed and filtered EEG. The upper tracing has a logarithmic amplitude display while the lower is linear. The duration of the trend recording is 3 h, but can be changed from 0.5 to 8 h. The raw EEG sample is 9 s and shows rhythmic high-amplitude activity at the time (05.02, shown below the trends) when the infant had a clinical seizure.

(b) The additional EEG sample shows the interictal EEG 22 min later (time 05.24)

2

Maturation of the electrocortical background

Interpretation of neonatal aEEG tracings is critically dependent on knowledge of the normal development of EEG from early preterm stages to the post-term period. This also includes EEG patterns in different stages of the sleep–wake cycle (active sleep, quiet sleep and wakefulness) at different gestational ages. When evaluating neonatal EEGs and aEEGs, the postconceptional age, i.e. the gestational age plus the postnatal age, must also be considered. Data from full polygraphic EEG studies have been summarized in this chapter[24–29] (Figures 2.1 and 2.2). With the advances in neonatal intensive care over the years, the survival rate for very premature infants has improved, and information on normal EEG development in this group has been added[29–31]. The overall quantitative development of EEG activity has also been studied with continuous recording using a more simplified four-channel tape recorder (Figure 2.3)[32–34].

With the aEEG technique it is possible to record cerebral activity for prolonged periods of time from full-term and preterm infants. The main features that can be extracted from such recordings concern the type of background activity in terms of continuous/discontinuous activity, interburst intervals, periodic variations in the background activity corresponding to sleep–wake cycling, and the occurrence of EEG seizure patterns (described in Chapter 4).

Information about hemispheric side asymmetries and synchrony, frequency content of EEG burst activity, occurrence of specific EEG features of clinical and prognostic significance such as delta brushes, positive rolandic sharp waves, other interictal sharp transients, etc. is not available, and full EEG recording is recommended for this purpose.

The mean interburst interval duration progressively decreases in normal infants from around 26 s at 21–22 weeks' gestation to around 13 s at 25–26 weeks[31]. At this stage of development the background activity is predominantly discontinuous (Figures 2.1 and 2.2)[29,30]. From 26 weeks' gestation onwards there is a gradual increase of the proportion of continuous EEG activity from around 10% to around 80% at full term (Figure 2.3a)[32]. During periods of discontinuous activity the mean interburst interval progressively decreases from around 13 s at 26 weeks' gestation to around 6 s at term (Figure 2.3b)[32]. A method for simplified classification of EEG into different categories of abnormality has been suggested by Ellison and colleagues[35].

Cyclic shifts of EEG activity, corresponding to variations of sleep and wakefulness, start to appear at around 26 weeks' gestation[29,30]. Between 32 and 35 weeks' gestation a *tracé discontinue* pattern is seen during quite sleep with decreasing interburst intervals gradually changing into a *tracé alternant* pattern at term. The main difference between these two variants of normal discontinuous EEG activity is the difference in amplitude of the EEG signal during the interburst intervals (Figure 2.2).

The normal developmental evolution of aEEG–CFM patterns in newborn infants of different gestational ages follows the EEG development (Figure 2.4)[36–38]. In parallel with EEG studies, cyclic variations corresponding with different sleep–wake states are found in the aEEG. The narrow trace in the aEEG represents more continuous activity during wakefulness or active sleep, and the periods of broad trace represent more discontinuous activity during quiet sleep (Figure 2.4). Correspondingly, in aEEG studies, sleep–wake cycling patterns have also been shown to emerge in records of preterm infants below 30 weeks' gestation (Figure 2.5)[39,40]. Corresponding to the gradual change from the *tracé discontinue* pattern in the preterm infant with very-low-voltage interburst activity to the *tracé alternant* pattern of the term infant, the minimum activity level of the CFM trace progressively increases[38] (Figures 2.4 and 2.6).

In full-term sick infants in neonatal intensive care, there is good agreement between aEEG and conventional EEG in the estimation of the degree of affection of the background activity and identification of seizure patterns[41–44]. Examples of abnormal background aEEG patterns are given in Figure 2.7.

The following classification of aEEG background patterns in full-term infants has been used for this Atlas[44,45]:

(1) The continuous normal voltage pattern (CNV; Figure 2.4) with maximum voltage 10–50 µV and with periods of increased variability due to quiet sleep;

(2) Mainly continuous normal voltage with periods of more discontinuous intermittent low voltage (no burst suppression) activity (DNV; Figure 2.7a);

(3) Discontinuous background pattern (burst suppression); periods of very low voltage (inactivity) intermixed with bursts of higher amplitude (Figure 2.7b);

(4) Continuous background pattern of very low voltage (around or below 5 µV; CVL; Figure 2.7c);

(5) Very low voltage, mainly inactive tracing with activity below 5 µV (FT; Figure 2.7d).

In very premature infants with *tracé discontinue* pattern with very-low-amplitude interburst activity it is difficult to differentiate a normal discontinuous background from burst suppression. Quantification of interburst interval or counting of bursts/h may give information in addition to mere visual judgement of the CFM trace (Figures 2.3 and 2.8).

In premature infants and in sick full-term infants with discontinuous background activity, arousing stimuli due to caregiving or diagnostic procedures often cause transient periods of continuous EEG activity. In the aEEG trace, this is seen as a period of increased minimum level of the trace (Figure 2.9b). This effect may be mistaken for a solitary period of seizure activity (see Chapter 4), and handling of the infant should always be noted in the trace record. Occasionally, activating stimulation may cause a more long-lasting shift from discontinuous to continuous activity (Figure 2.9a). In more healthy term infants with the CNV pattern, arousing stimulation causes a transient increase of low-amplitude high-frequency EEG components and a decrease of low-frequency components (see Figure 1.1). This does not usually produce a discernible shift in the aEEG trace presented on a logarithmic or semilogarithmic scale. This is presumably the reason why the presence or absence of arousal responses in the aEEG trace has not been proven to have a significant prognostic significance[46]. Sometimes, frequent care procedures in premature infants seem to cause a deterioration of a discontinuous pattern, rather than an activation effect (Figure 2.9c).

Soon after its development, CFM was used for the monitoring of general anesthesia[5]. In adult subjects, initiation of anesthesia causes an increase in rhythmic EEG activity and an increase in the CFM trace. Only with progressively deep levels of anesthesia were DNV, burst suppression and electrocerebral inactivity recorded. In light anesthesia, painful stimuli cause abrupt increases of activity together with signs of muscle activity in the impedance trace. Drugs with sedative and depressing effects on the brain may also affect the aEEG background and increase the amount of discontinuous activity in preterm and ill full-term infants[47,48]. In infants with CNV or DNV patterns, administration of a sedative often produces a shift to a burst-suppression pattern, and in infants with an established burst-suppression pattern the burst density often decreases (Figure 2.8). Our impression is that the effect of sedatives is partly due to the dose given, and partly due to the degree of the metabolic derangement of the brain as a result of asphyxia or other pathological conditions. The effects are often transient, and it is of paramount importance to document the time of initiation of treatment and the administered doses on the aEEG trace in order to avoid misinterpretations (Figures 2.10, 2.11 and 2.12).

Administration of surfactant often causes a profound and transient depression of the background activity, as seen in Figure 2.13[49]. The mechanism for this effect is still unknown. It is important to differentiate this effect from other more serious causes of sudden deterioration of the background activity, such as the pneumothorax illustrated in Figure 2.14[50].

Maturational development of continuous EEG activity

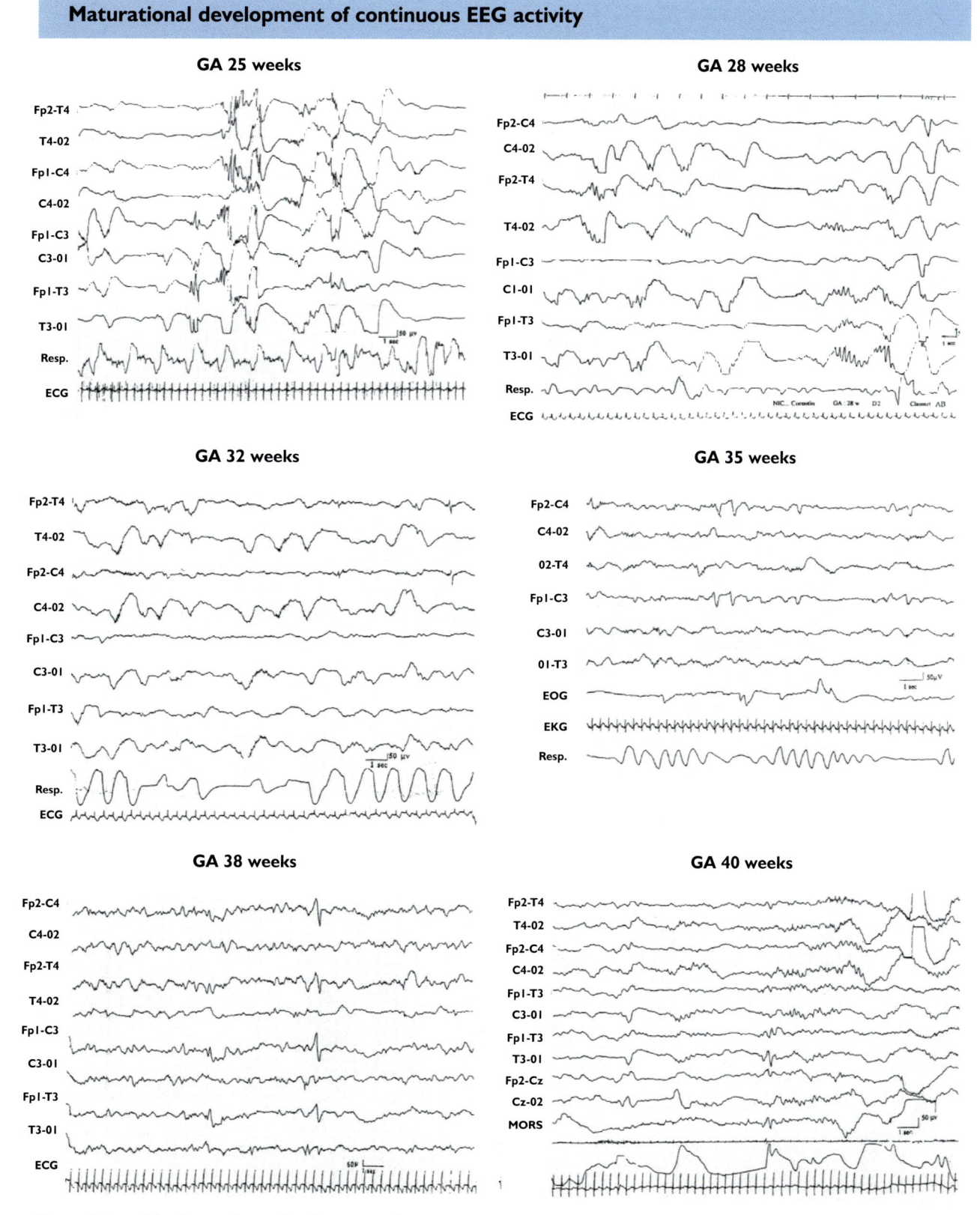

Figure 2.1   The figure shows development of continuous EEG activity, representing active sleep and/or periods of wakefulness, at different gestational ages (GA). Reproduced from reference 29 with permission. At 25 weeks' gestational age the EEG is predominantly discontinuous with only brief (< 60 s) periods of continuous activity. From 28 weeks' gestational age the periods of continuous activity become longer and more frequent. From 32 weeks' gestation and onwards, active sleep and wakefulness stages show a continuous EEG pattern

Maturational development of EEG during quiet sleep

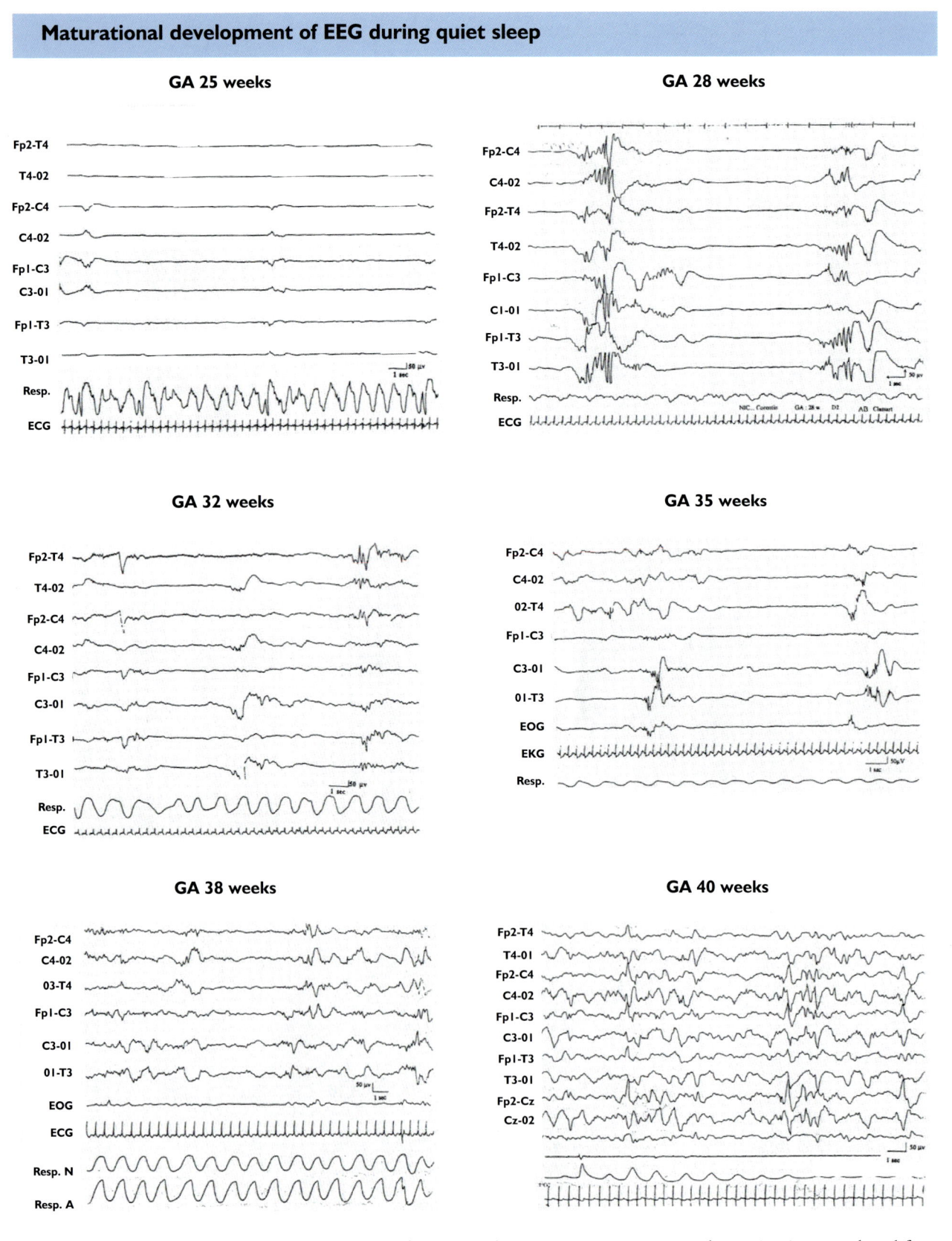

Figure 2.2 Examples of polygraphic EEG records in quiet sleep at increasing gestational ages (GA). Reproduced from reference 29 with permission. At 25 and 28 weeks' gestation the trace is very discontinuous. At 32 and 35 weeks' gestational age, a *tracé discontinue* pattern is seen with decreasing interburst intervals gradually changing into a *tracé alternant* pattern at term

Maturational development of aEEG

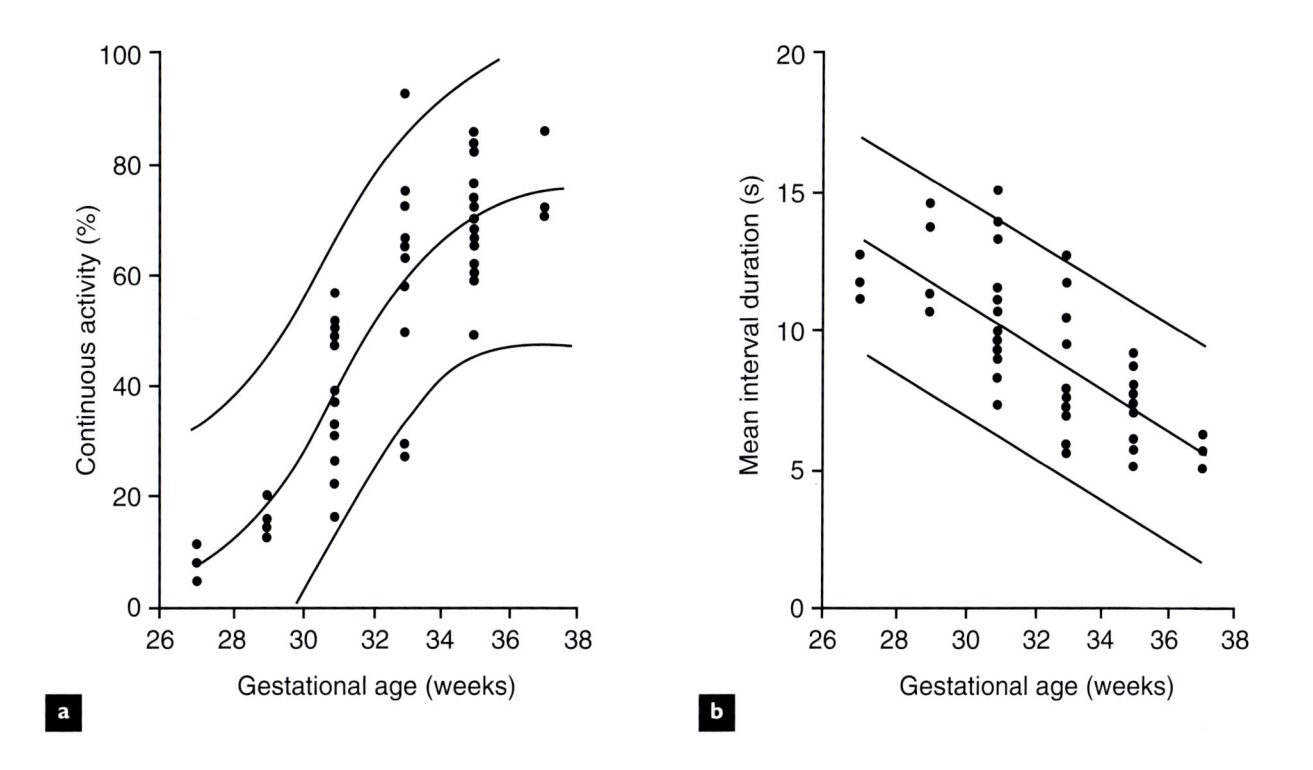

Figure 2.3   (a) Percentage increase of continuous EEGs from gestational age 26–37 weeks from around 10% to over 80%. From reference 32 with permission.   (b) Development of mean interburst interval duration with gestational age. Measurements were made from the most discontinuous quiet-sleep part of each of 45 recordings in infants of 26–37 weeks' gestational age using a four-channel Oxford Medilog recorder. From reference 32 with permission

The aEEG examples in this Atlas were recorded with a paper speed of 6 cm/h, unless stated otherwise. Although the scales in the presented figures differ, 6 cm/h corresponds to a time-scale with 10 min between the vertical lines in the recordings.

Normal development of aEEG in infant from 31 to 37 weeks' gestation

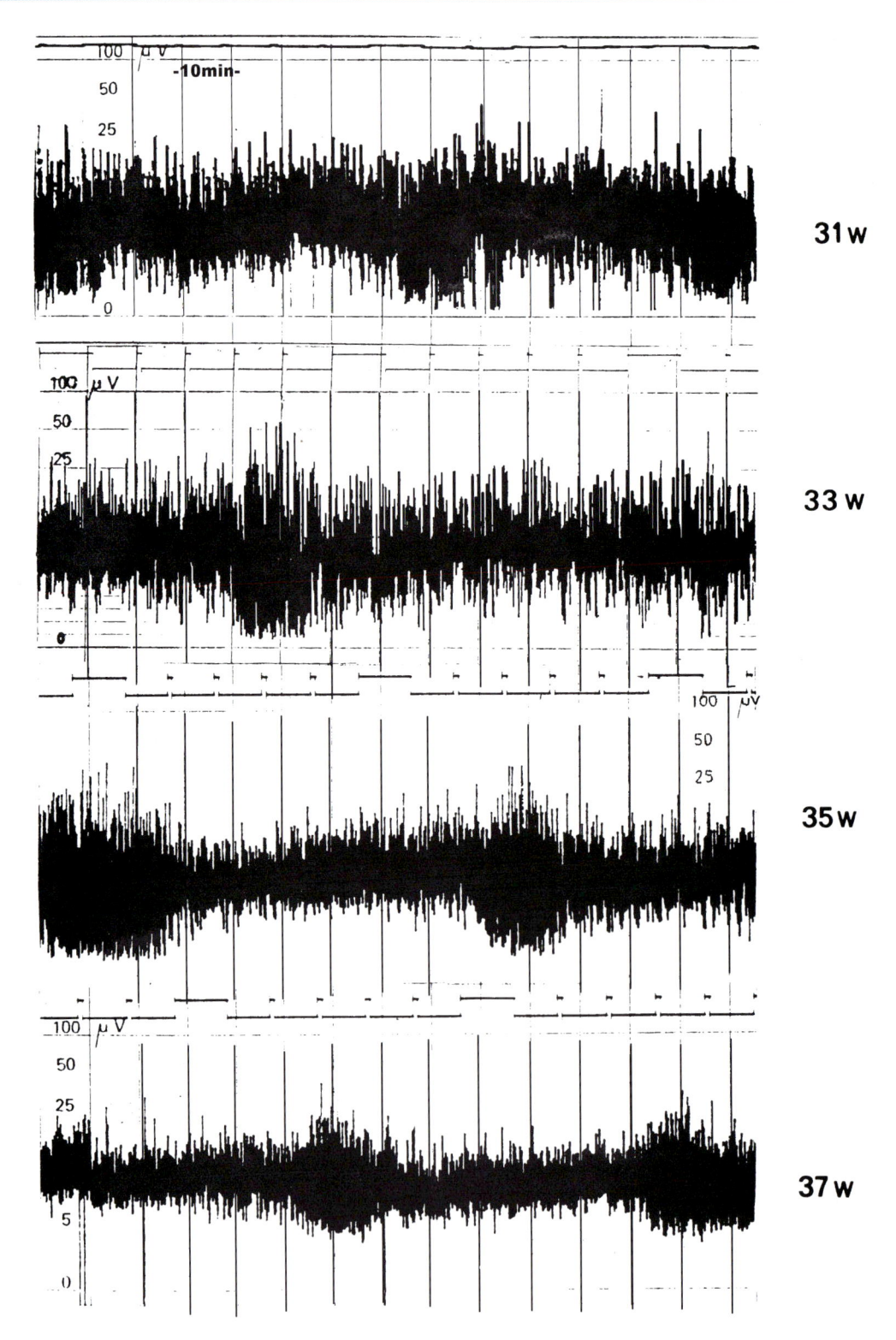

Figure 2.4 Consecutive recording of an aEEG by CFM in an infant of 30 weeks' gestation from 31 to 37 weeks of age. Reproduced from reference 38 with permission. Periods of quiet sleep with discontinuous EEG activity show up in the aEEG record as periods with large min–max amplitude fluctuations as compared with less fluctuations during periods with continuous EEG (active sleep and wakefulness). Note transient shift of minimum amplitudes during quiet sleep close to zero at 31 and 33 weeks (*tracé discontinue*) to levels around 5 µV at 37 weeks (*tracé alternant*)

Cyclic changes in background activity in extremely preterm infants

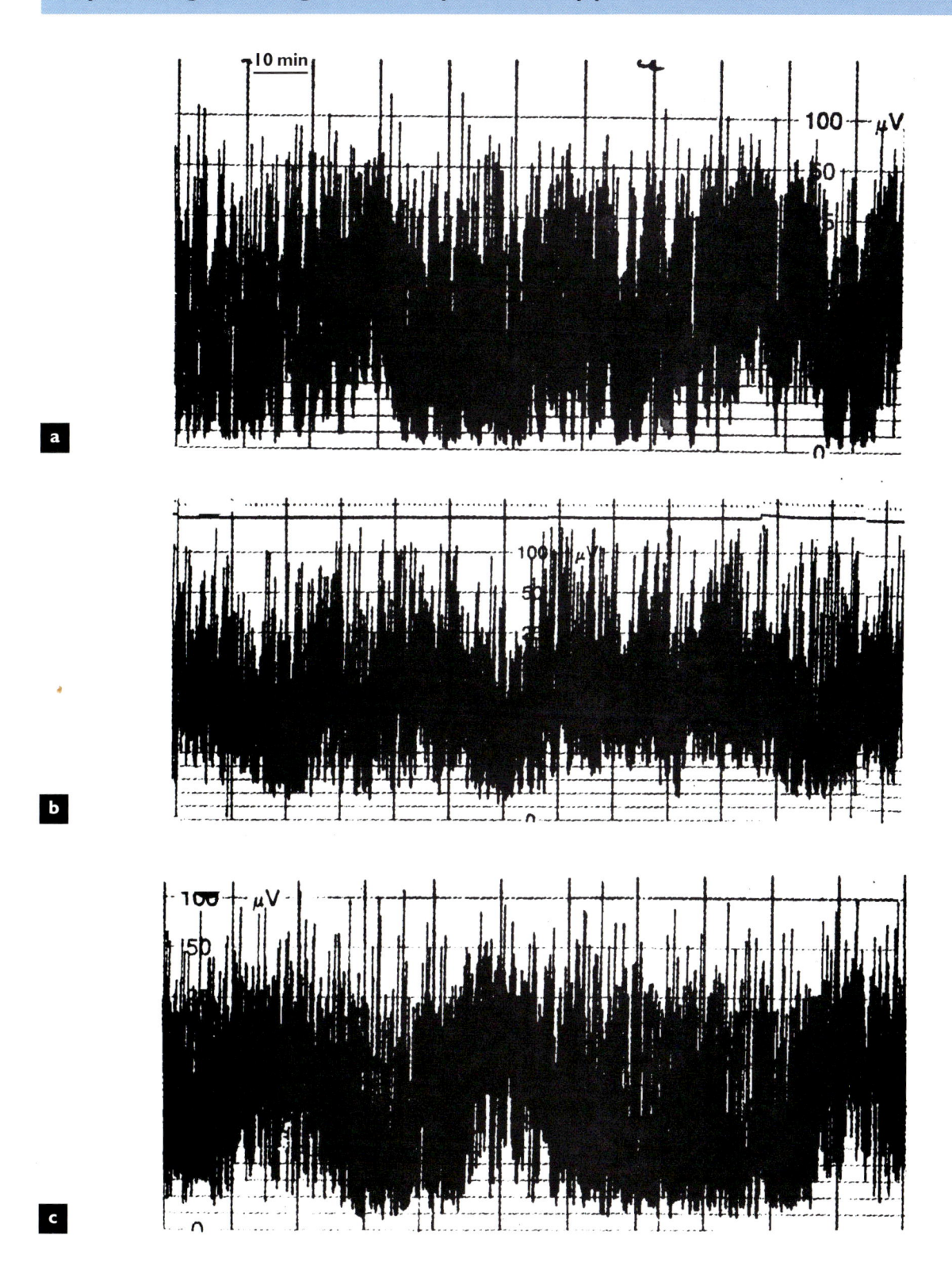

Figure 2.5   Cyclic changes of background activity, in both amplitude and continuity, resembling sleep–wake cycling can also be demonstrated by aEEG in extremely preterm infants. (a, gestational age 26 weeks + 21 days; b, gestational age 24 weeks + 6 days; c, gestational age 25 weeks + 7 days). Reproduced from reference 40 with permission

Normal variations in CFM amplitude in different age groups

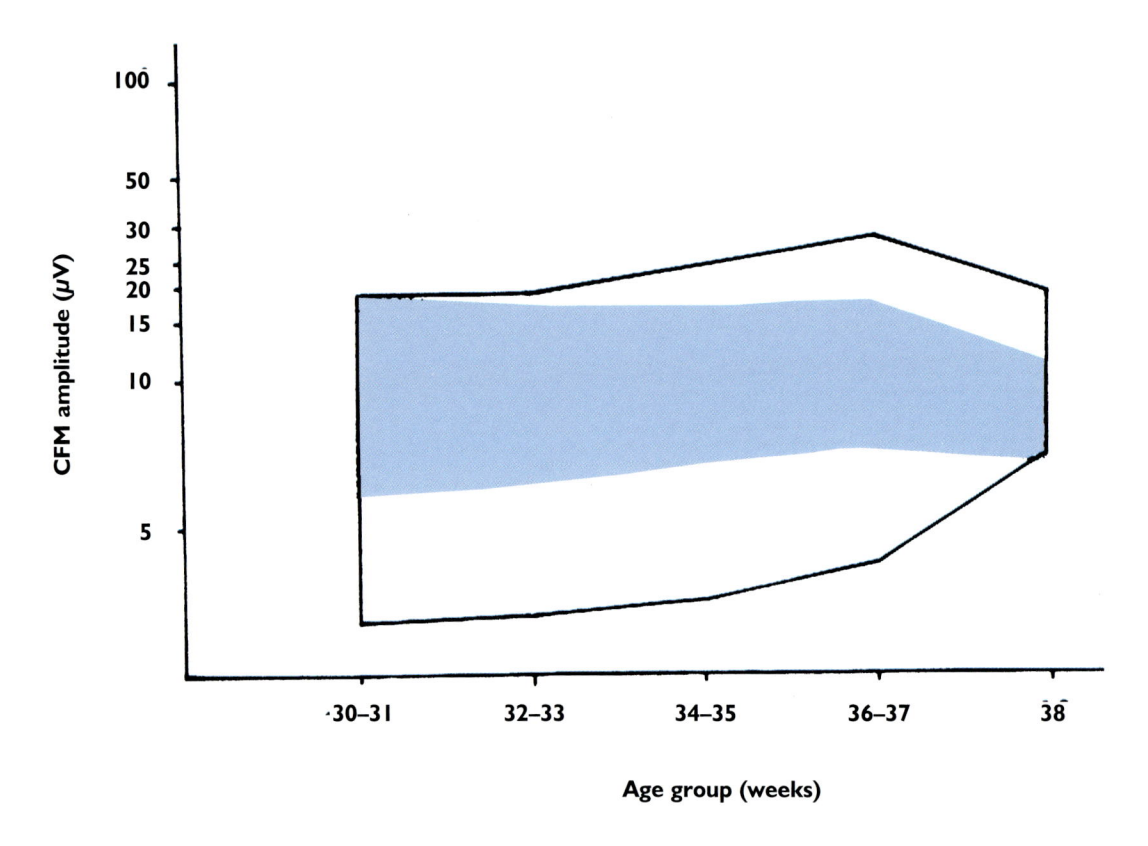

Figure 2.6   Normal variations in CFM amplitude in different age groups. The white area shows the variation of the broadest band width (corresponding to quiet sleep), the colored area the narrowest band width (corresponding to active sleep and wakefulness). From reference 38 with permission

Figure 2.7 *opposite*   Each of these four tracings shows 4–4.5 h of electrocortical background activity.

At the beginning of trace (a) the CFM has been calibrated. Accurate setting of the zero level of the amplitude is important for proper identification of a flat trace, as compared with a low voltage continuous (CLV) activity, and for differentiating burst suppression from discontinuous normal voltage (DNV) activity.

(a) A discontinuous background pattern with normal voltage (DNV). During the recording the background changes to a continuous normal voltage (CNV) pattern.

(b) A stable burst-suppression background with no changes due to, for example, handling. The burst density is rather dense, i.e. around 100–150 bursts/h, as compared to the relatively sparse burst density (58/h) following administration of diazepam in Figure 2.8.

(c) A continuous but extremely low voltage pattern (CLV) with no variability. The short and relatively high-amplitude changes (up to 25 µV) occurring in the middle of the tracing are probably movement artefacts or other artefacts.

(d) A mainly inactive, i.e. flat tracing, although in the beginning a few bursts of activity could also be said to represent a very sparse burst-suppression pattern (burst activity with 1–20 min intervals)

Abnormal background patterns in the full-term infant

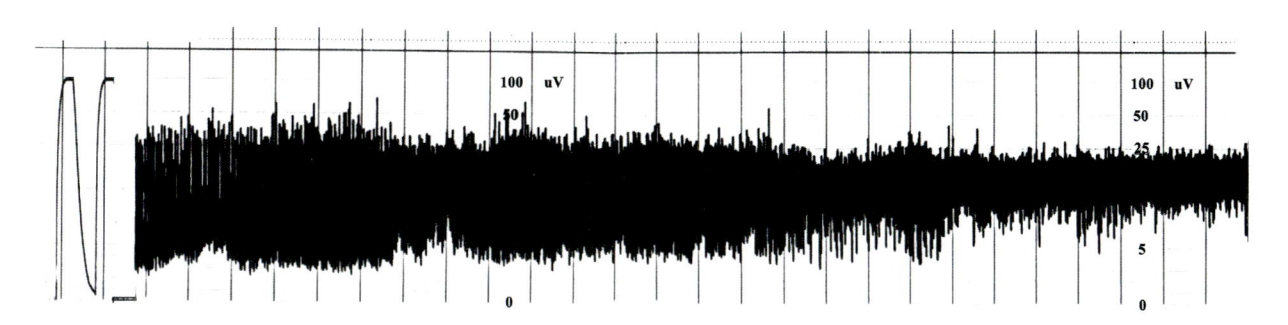

a

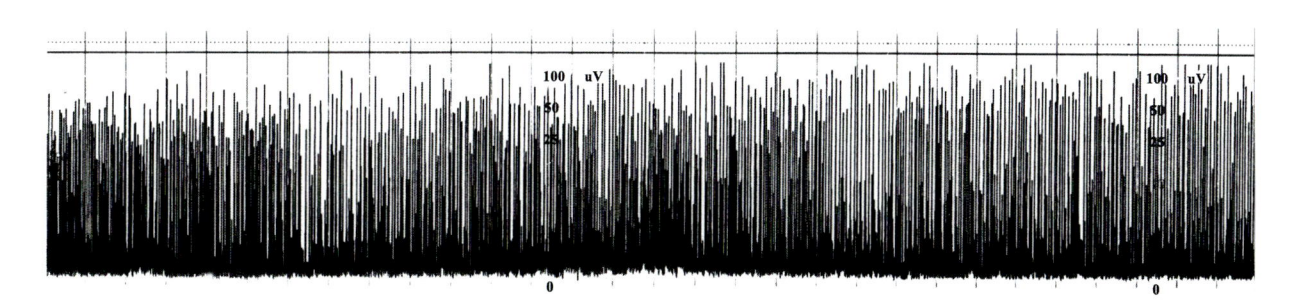

b

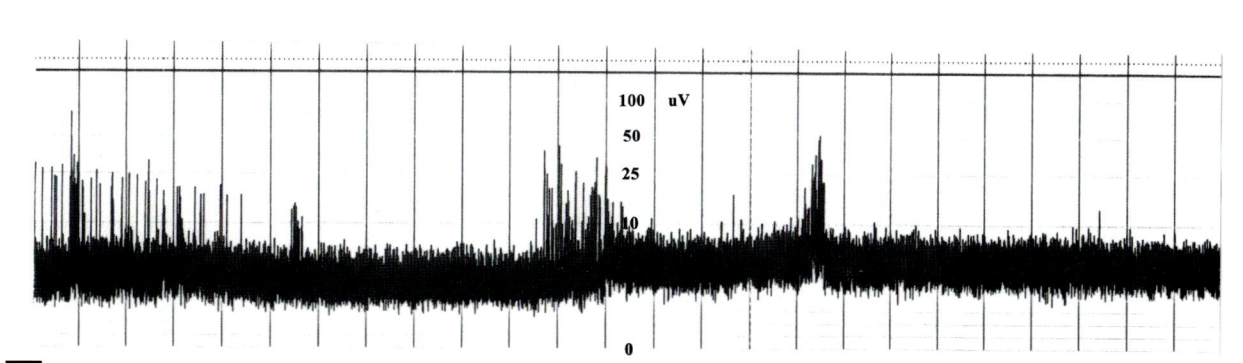

c

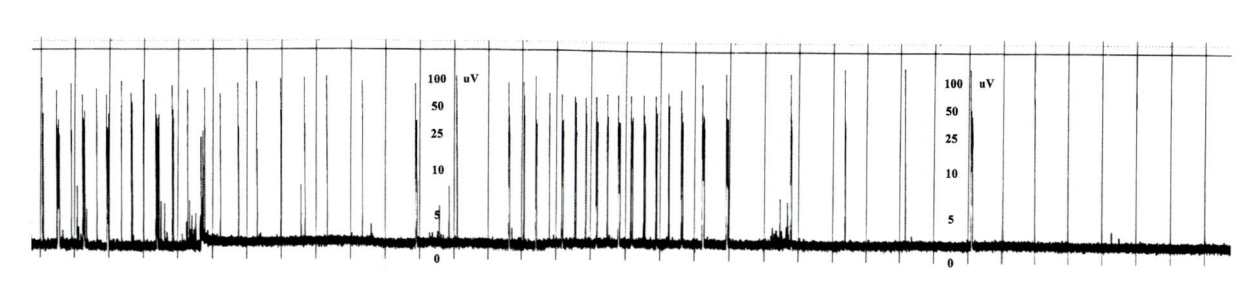

d

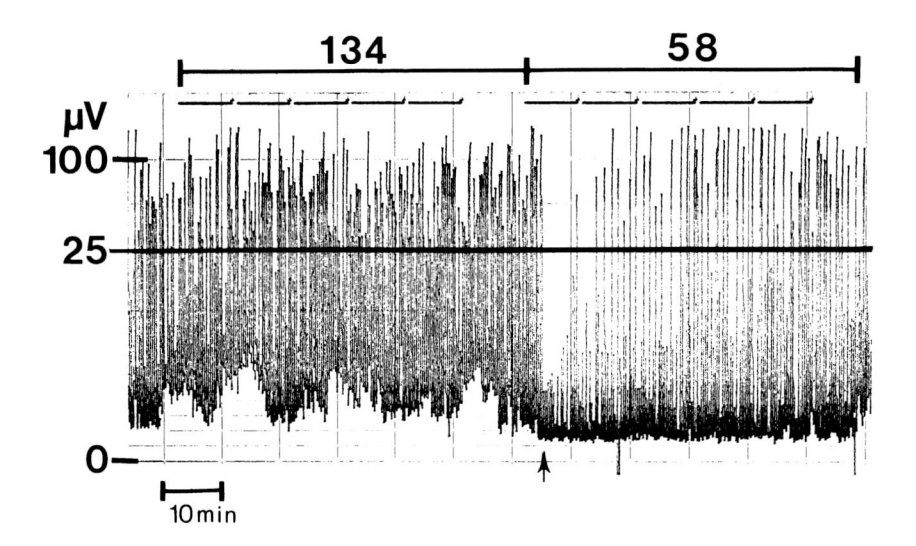

Figure 2.8 Decrease in burst/h following the administration of diazepam (arrow) in a premature infant

Arousal in a full-term infant

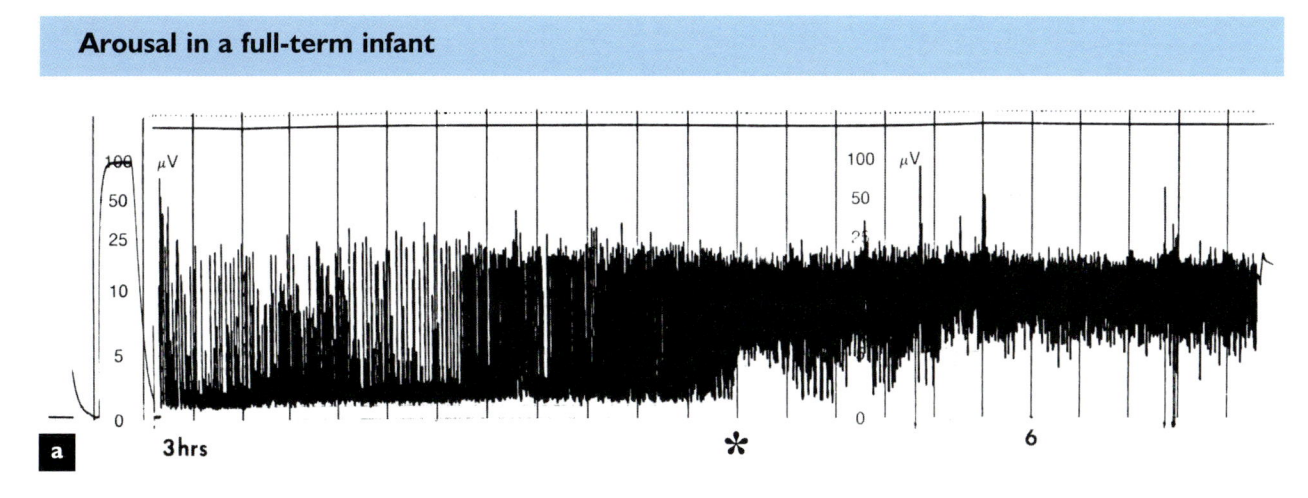

Figure 2.9 (a) This male infant was born at 40 weeks' gestation, following a vaginal breech delivery complicated by asphyxia. He was immediately resuscitated and intubated. Phenobarbitone was administered prophylactically at 1 h of age. He developed persistent pulmonary hypertension and required ventilation for 14 days.

The aEEG was started at 3 h of age. Initially, there was a burst-suppression pattern. The background recovered slowly and continuously during the first 2 h of recording. The recovery shows as increased burst density and a subtle, but continuous, increase in the minimum amplitude. At 5 h of age a more abrupt change to a CNV pattern occurred, probably due to arousal when evoked potentials were done (at asterisk)

Transient changes during caregiving

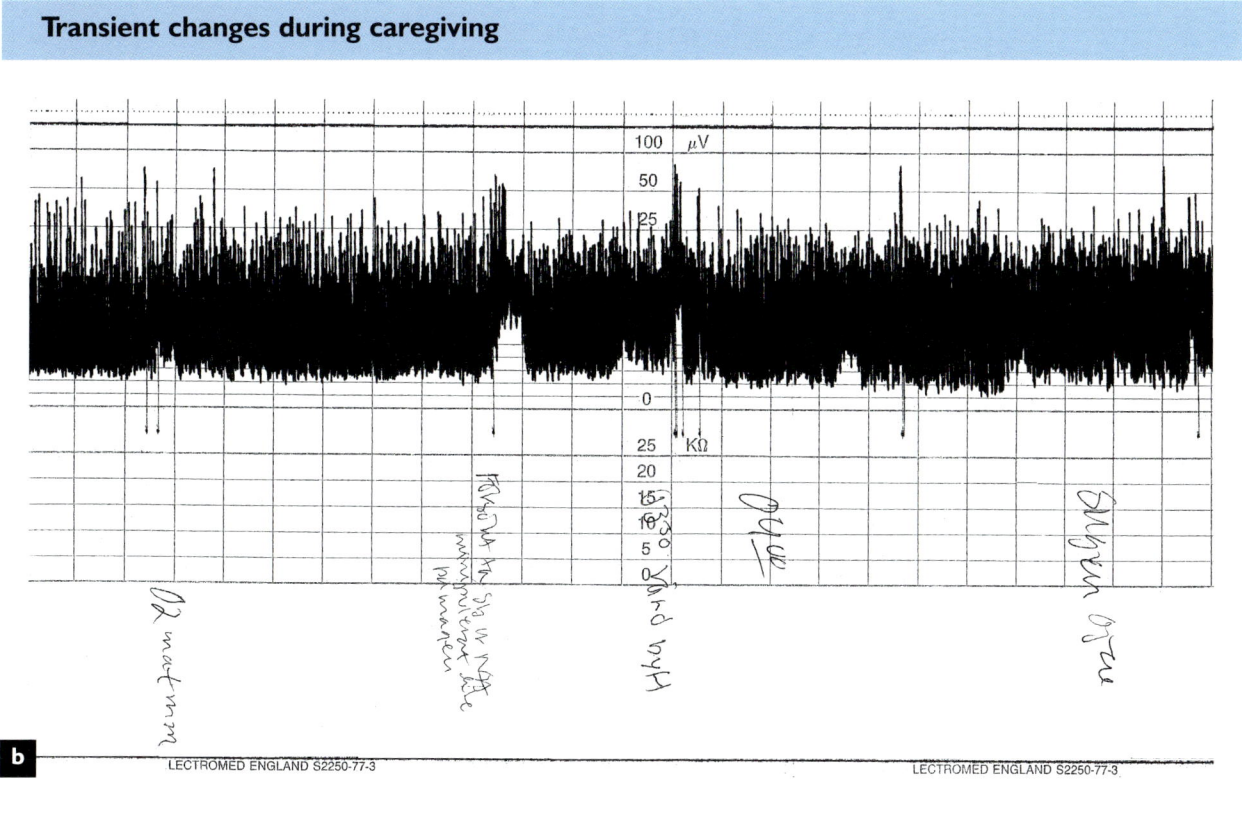

Figure 2.9 continued (b) This full-term infant with moderate HIE had an abnormal discontinuous aEEG background corresponding with a burst-suppression pattern. Concomitant with caregiving procedures (written below the trace) and representing arousals due to the handling, transient increases in the minimum amplitude of the aEEG can be seen. A subtle change of the general background activity, which becomes increasingly continuous, can also be seen. The improvement is mainly due to a larger variability of the minimum amplitude of the recording, indicating more continuous activity although of quite low amplitude

Effect of frequent caregiving in an extremely preterm infant

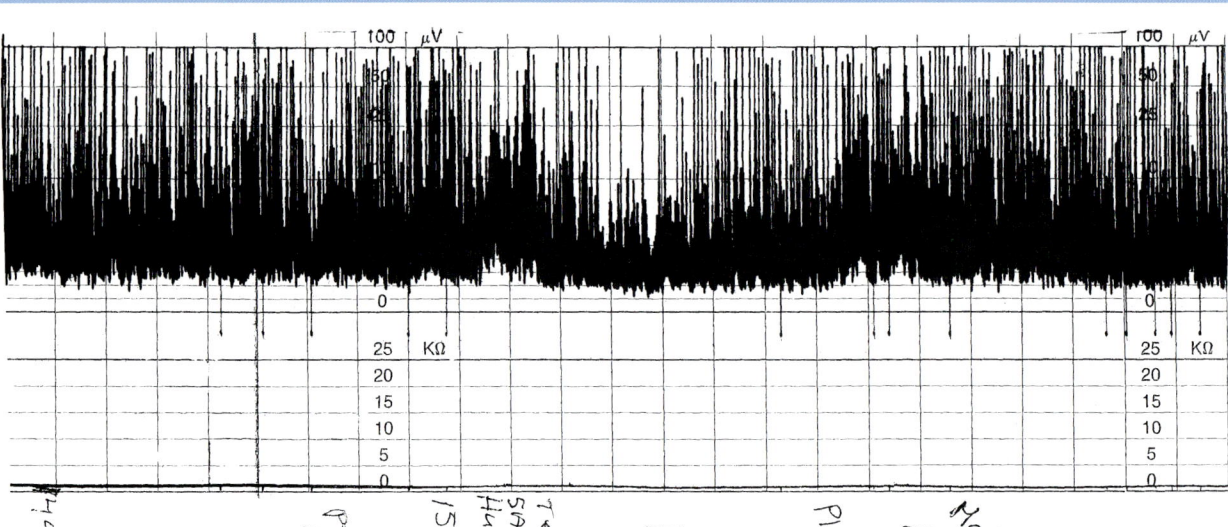

Figure 2.9 continued (c) This infant of 25 weeks' gestation was stable on mechanical ventilation. He had aEEG monitoring as a clinical routine during intensive care. The aEEG background in this 4-h tracing can be considered as normal for the gestation although a cyclical pattern, resembling sleep–wake cycling, can sometimes be seen in spontaneously breathing infants. Following several caregiving procedures (clinical notes below the trace), the burst density transiently decreased in the middle of the tracing. This reaction is not unusual in extremely preterm infants, and could be a sign of 'cerebral exhaustion' as a response to excessive stimulation

Transient cerebral deterioration during endotracheal suctioning

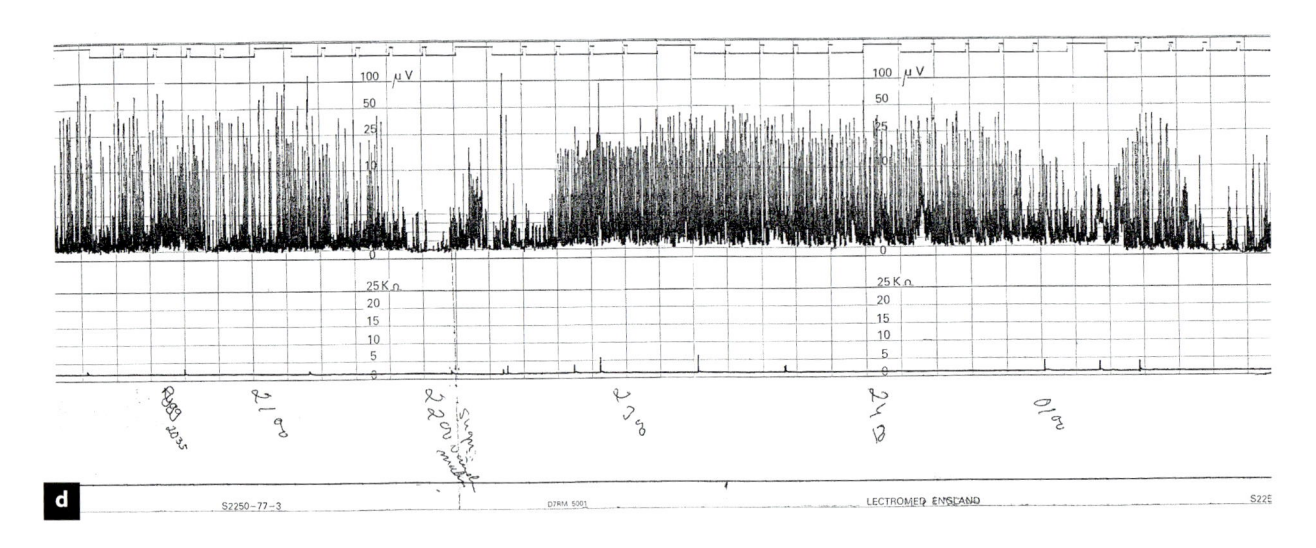

Figure 2.9 continued (d) This was an unstable, extremely preterm infant with severe RDS. The initial aEEG background shows a burst-suppression pattern with relatively low burst density. In the middle of the tracing, the endotracheal tube was suctioned which also resulted in a transient severe depression of the aEEG background. The background activity recovered but deteriorated again when the infant developed a massive pulmonary hemorrhage and died at the end of the recording

Effect of midazolam in a full-term asphyxiated infant

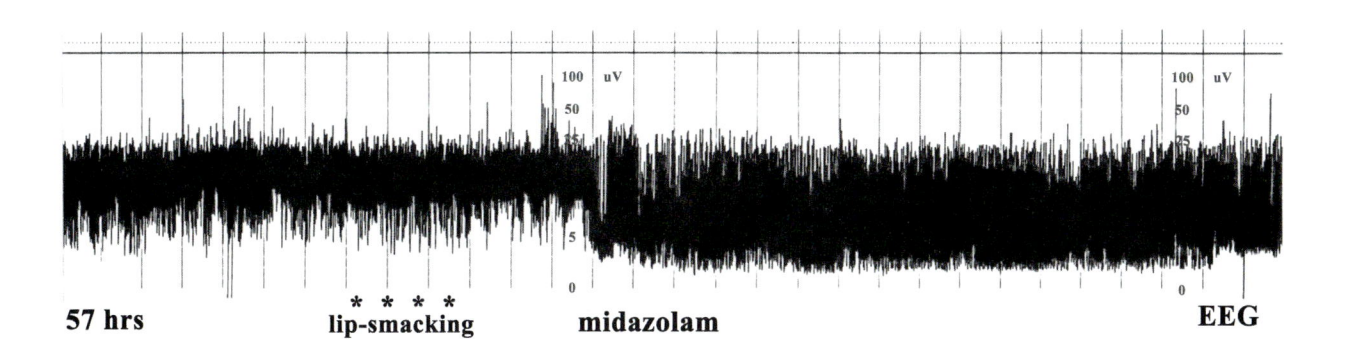

Figure 2.10 This male infant was born at home following a normal pregnancy. The delivery was complicated by shoulder dystocia. He had a very poor start with Apgar scores 0, 1 and 2 at 1, 5 and 10 min, respectively, but then he recovered quickly. His cranial ultrasound scan, as well as the MRI performed at the end of the first week, were normal. At 18 months of age he showed normal neurodevelopmental outcome with a developmental quotient of 110.

The aEEG shows a DNV background pattern but no sleep–wake cycling. The infant had a period with lip-smacking (marked by asterisks) but without any clear epileptic seizure activity in the aEEG. A loading dose of midazolam (0.05 mg/kg in 20 min) resulted in a change of the background to a burst-suppression pattern. A standard EEG, performed a few hours later, also showed burst suppression. Recovery of the background activity was seen the following day.

This example shows the depressing effect on the aEEG background that can occur following a loading dose of midazolam

Effect of phenobarbitone

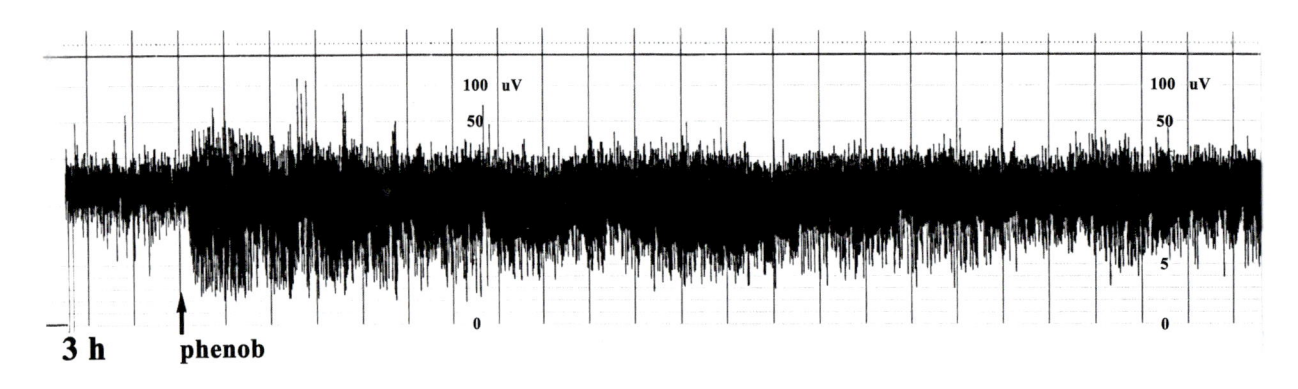

3 h   phenob

a

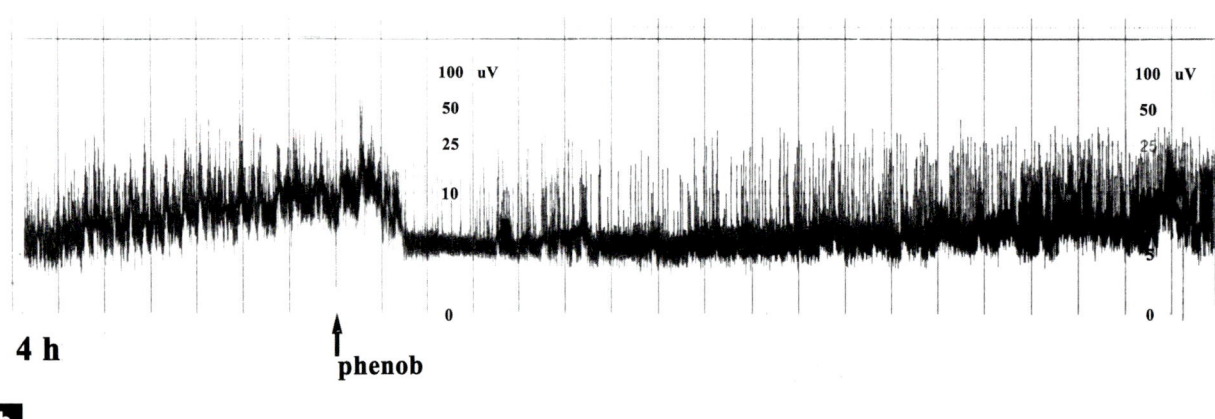

4 h   phenob

b

Figure 2.11   The effect of a loading dose of phenobarbitone (20 mg/kg intravenously) is shown in two full-term infants.

(a) This infant had mild HIE, and the aEEG starting at 3 h showed a CNV pattern. Phenobarbitone (phenob) was given prophylactically (at arrow) and changed the background to a more discontinuous but normal voltage (DNV) pattern, as reflected by the lower minimum amplitude. The background activity recovered over the following 4 h.

(b) In the second infant with moderate HIE a low-voltage 'saw-tooth' pattern, corresponding with recurrent epileptic seizure activity, was present at the beginning of the recording. After phenobarbitone (phenob; arrow), the electrographic seizure pattern ceased and the background became flat for almost 30 min. Then a low-voltage burst-suppression pattern returned with increasing burst density and some suspected epileptic seizure activity. There was a drift of the baseline; the minimum level of the aEEG activity should (probably) be lower than 4–5 µV. The baseline drift is difficult to explain. The output from the aEEG is very sensitive to low-voltage activity, which could also be extracranial, and such baseline drifts mainly occur in patients with very-low-voltage aEEG activity.

Phenobarbitone may affect the electrocortical background, but the degree of the effect on the aEEG is dependent on the dose and on the severity of the underlying condition

Effect of pethidine and morphine in preterm infants

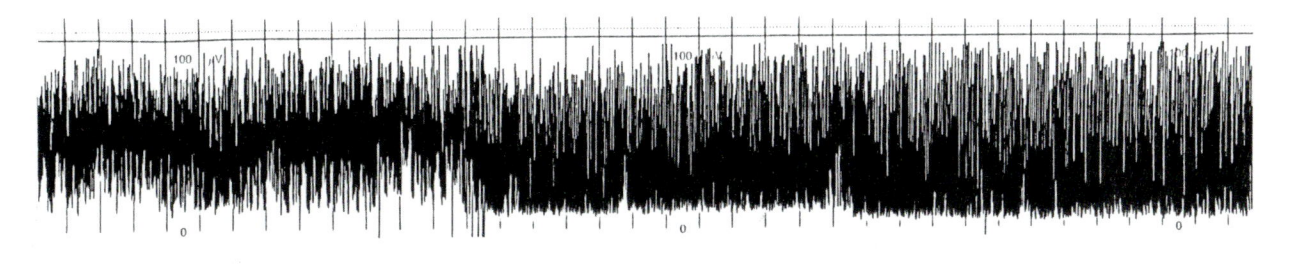

↑ pethidine

a

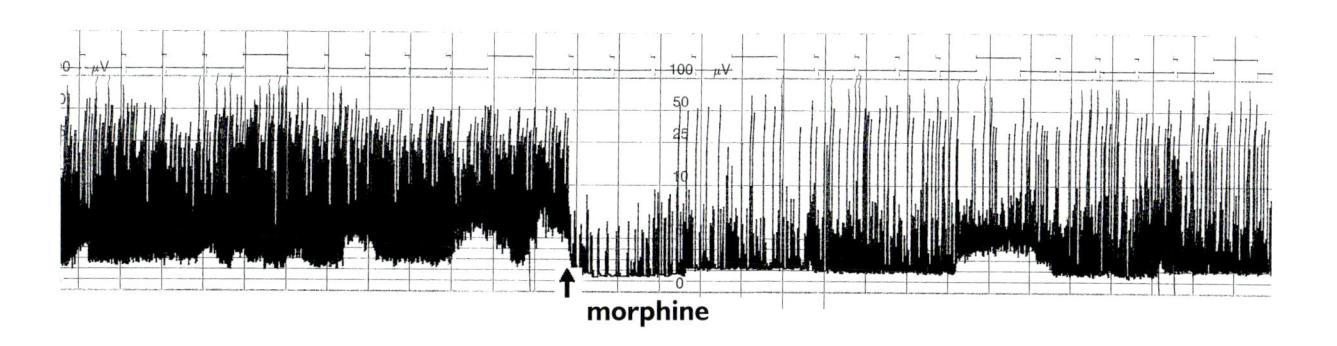

↑ morphine

b

Figure 2.12   (a) This recording was performed on the first day of life in a preterm infant of 29 weeks' gestational age (GA). Following initiation of ventilatory support, a loading dose of pethidine (1 mg intravenously) was given for sedation. The variable background, containing both continuous and discontinuous activity, which is appropriate for an infant of this gestation, immediately became more discontinuous and changed to a burst-suppression pattern.

(b) This was a female infant of 30 weeks' gestation with severe Rhesus immunization. A blood-exchange transfusion had just been performed and she was stable on mechanical ventilation. She received intravenous morphine (at the arrow) for sedation. The initially discontinuous aEEG background, showing some baseline variability and considered normal for the gestation, was immediately affected and became severely depressed and almost inactive for 20 min following the morphine. The electrocortical background recovered as a burst-suppression pattern with increasing burst density over the following 2 h. Such a marked reaction to morphine is uncommon, but tells us that this infant had a certain degree of cerebral fragility. She survived and was discharged with no signs of cerebral injury. In a study on electrocortical responses during blood exchange transfusions, only small changes occurred in the aEEG amplitude and seemed to be associated with changes in mean arterial blood pressure[51]

Effect of surfactant

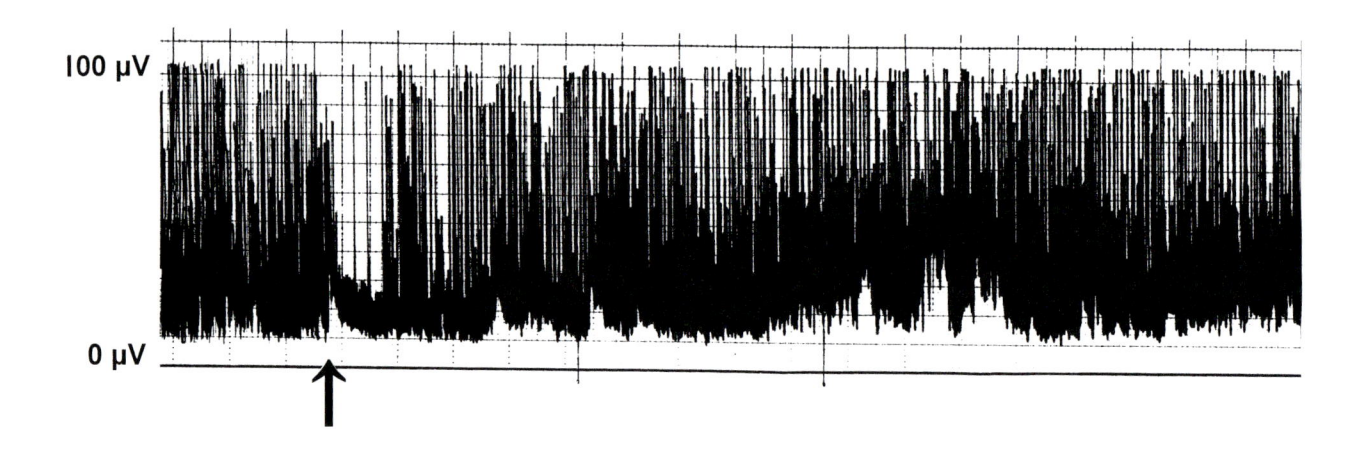

Figure 2.13   In this preterm infant of 26 weeks' gestation, surfactant was administered intratracheally as a bolus (at the arrow). The discontinuous burst-suppression background immediately became flat for 10 min before cerebral activity returned to the previous background pattern. This reaction to surfactant is very common, but the mechanisms are not understood[49]

Pneumothorax

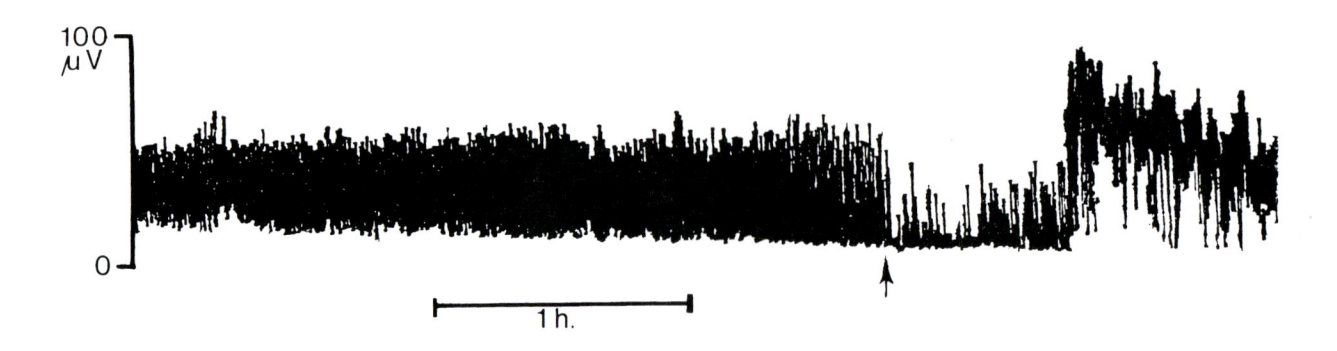

Figure 2.14   This aEEG example is from a full-term infant with severe meconium aspiration who developed a pneumothorax. He was on mechanical ventilation but was difficult to oxygenate. In the beginning of the recording the aEEG background was mainly continuous. During the following 3 h there was a gradual depression of the background activity, which changed to a discontinuous burst-suppression pattern. A sudden deterioration of cerebral activity occurred at the arrow, and the aEEG background was mainly flat for the following 40 min. The aEEG deterioration took place simultaneously with a severe deterioration in oxygenation due to a pneumothorax. The infant was resuscitated but died at the end of the recording. The aEEG activity that can be seen during the last 20–30 min is due to movement artefacts. Reproduced from reference 50 with permission

3

Pitfalls and caveats

In this chapter we discuss some pitfalls and caveats encountered with aEEG monitoring, and especially the CFM, in neonatal intensive care. In contrast to digital EEG monitoring devices, the CFM systems do not allow us to inspect the raw EEG. The unprocessed EEG is by far the best way of disclosing extracerebral artefact sources in unexpected trend patterns. As for all EEG recording, careful control of electrode impedances is important for avoiding artefacts. The CFM equipment has a second recording channel for impedance monitoring (see Figure 3.5) and an indicator lamp on the panel signalling when impedance is in excess of $20 \, k\Omega$. The preferred impedance during recording is below $5 \, k\Omega$.

A temporary artefact exceeding $800 \, \mu V$ peak-to-peak will cause a cut-out of both recording channels and illuminate the indicator lamp (see Figure 3.5). Periodic or continuous artefacts below this threshold level, which could directly interfere with the EEG signal and affect the interpretation, are more difficult to reveal. Repeated gasping or other repeated motor activity may be misinterpreted as discontinuous aEEG patterns (Figures 3.1 and 7.13 in Chapter 7) and should be noted directly on the recording trace. Administration of a muscle relaxant may solve the problem in mechanically ventilated infants. The NICU is a very EEG-'unfriendly' environment with several electrical and mechanical sources of artefacts[52]. High-frequency ventilation usually adds to the input signal with an upward shift of the baseline (Figure 3.2). Shifting of the head position possibly establishing an unintentional mechanical contact with the underlying pillow may allow an extracranial artefact to be added to the input (Figure 3.3). Notes made directly on the record trace documenting handling and care procedures of the patient and changes of head position are of great value in the *post hoc* evaluation of the record.

Several examples are given here and in later chapters (Figures 3.6, 5.6, 5.9, 5.11 and 7.18) of unexplained upward shifts of the baseline level in CFM records expected to be burst-suppression pattern or flat. It is often impossible to trace the source of the signal responsible, often only a few microvolts in amplitude. Intracranial sources, such as a very-low-amplitude continuous cerebral rhythm or epileptiform activity are feasible, as well as pick-up from extracranial sources such as ECG or pulsative mechanical movements. Due to the very low amplitude, standard EEG is often unhelpful in this situation. Close collaboration with clinical neurophysiologists is an advantage and will probably improve the quality of the clinical monitoring.

In cases of lateralized hemispheric lesions (Figures 3.7, 3.8, 6.6 and 7.17) the background activity as well as epileptiform seizure activity may be quite asymmetrical. A single-channel biparietal recording would then present a weighted average of the background activity. Although seizure patterns, even when focal (see Figure 6.7), are usually discernible in the standard biparietal lead, very focal seizure patterns may be missed (Figure 3.8)[44]. When lateralized lesions are suspected, an early diagnostic standard EEG is recommended. Based on topographic information obtained, the position of the recording monitoring electrodes may be changed. When available, a two-channel monitoring of activity from each hemisphere may be of value.

- The aEEG should always be calibrated before each recording;

- When calibrated, the zero level is the most important and this should be correct;

- During long-term recordings the aEEG should be calibrated every 24 h;

- The impedance during recording should be kept below 5 kΩ;

- High-frequency ventilation can make the aEEG recording unreliable;

- Do not apply needle electrodes above fontanelles or sutures;

- Do not apply electrodes over cephalic hematoma or other local abnormalities on the skull;

- Do not position the electrodes in direct contact with bedding;

- Frequent clinical notes on the tracing will facilitate later interpretation;

- At least one conventional EEG should be performed in most infants with aEEG monitoring.

Effect of gasping

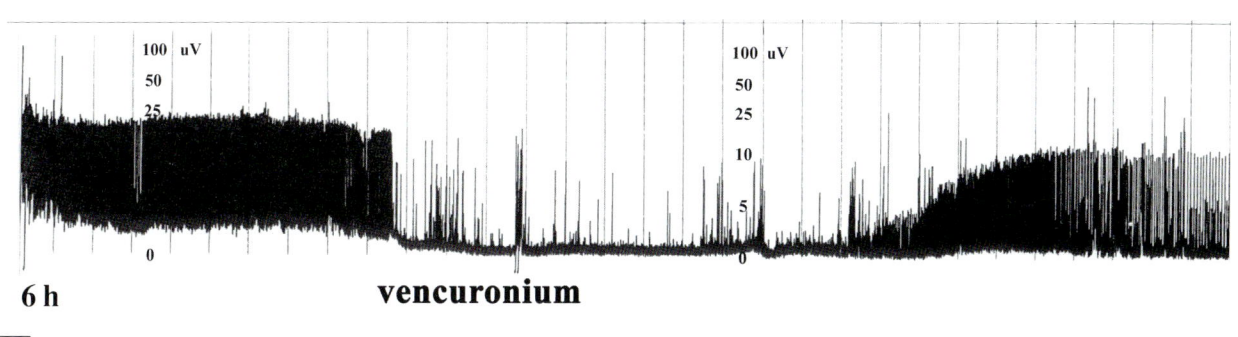

6 h   vencuronium

a

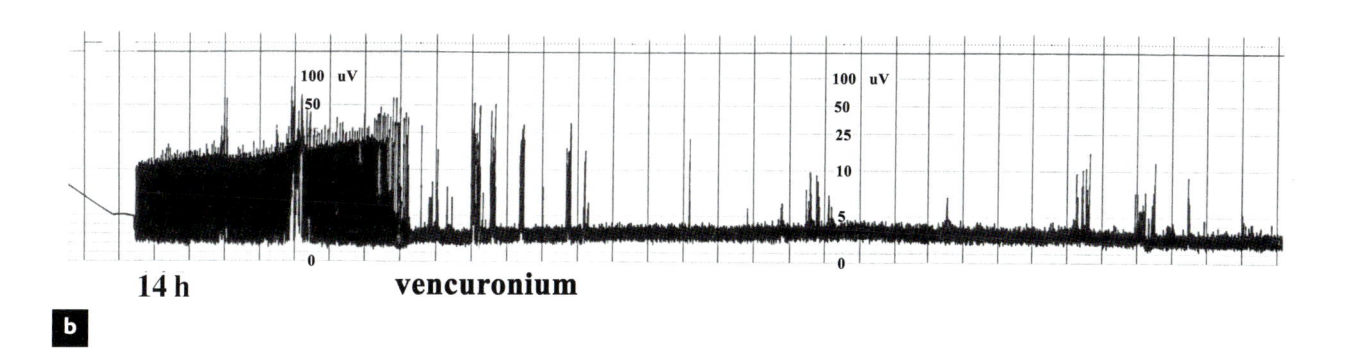

14 h   vencuronium

b

Figure 3.1 (a) This aEEG tracing is from a full-term infant with severe HIE. The infant was continuously gasping on the ventilator. The initial aEEG can be interpreted as a burst-suppression pattern. However, following a loading dose of vencuronium, a muscle relaxant, the aEEG background became flat. After about 2 h, the effect of the muscle-paralyzing agent was wearing off. The gasping started again, and in the aEEG again a burst-suppression-like background was seen. The impedance was low (zero) all the time. Reproduced from reference 53 with permission.

(b) The lower tracing from another severely asphyxiated infant is very similar except that a continuous infusion of vencuronium was given. There was no return of gasping and the aEEG remained flat.

This artefact is rare, but should be excluded when severely brain-injured infants on mechanical ventilation are gasping and the aEEG shows burst suppression. On these occasions a loading dose of a muscle-paralyzing agent can be used to make interpretation of the aEEG more reliable. A standard EEG would also reveal the artefact

Effect of high-frequency ventilation

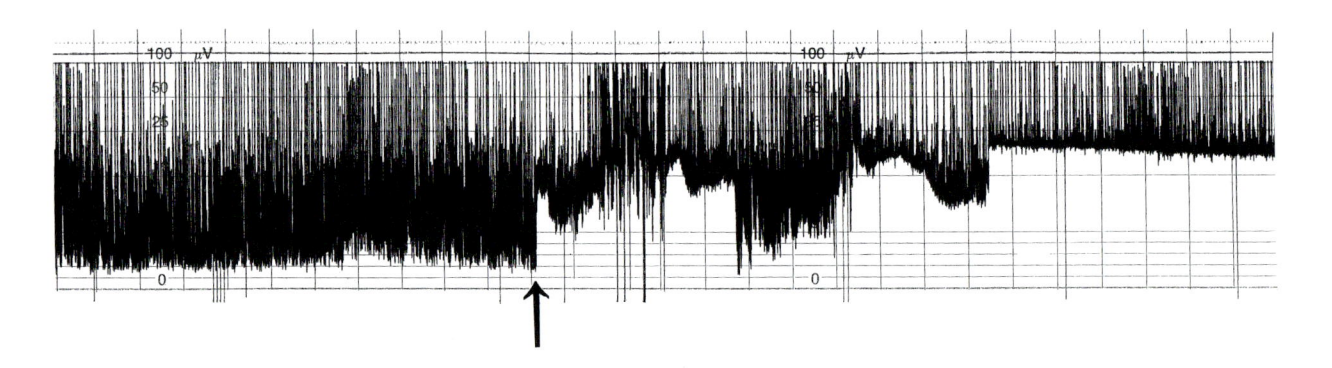

Figure 3.2 This is a common artefact that makes the aEEG less reliable during high-frequency ventilation. This infant of 25 weeks' gestation with severe respiratory distress syndrome needed high-frequency ventilation. He had aEEG for routine clinical monitoring. The high-frequency ventilation, starting at the arrow, resulted in a drift of the baseline that made the recording very difficult and unreliable to interpret. The discontinuous background can still be seen after the start of high-frequency ventilation but other changes, e.g. variations in the background or epileptic seizure activity, may be impossible to detect

Effect of head position

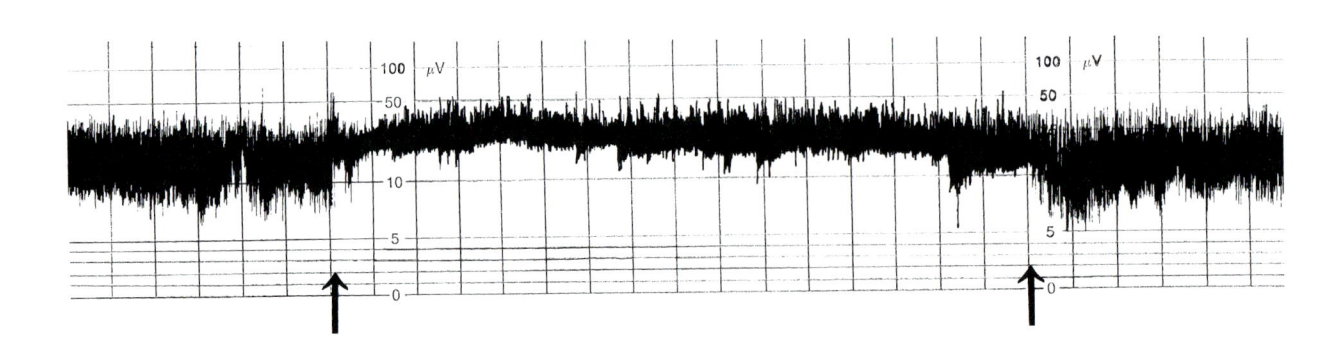

Figure 3.3 An optimal biparietal position of the electrodes is not always possible due, for example, to cephalic hematoma or caregiving. However, if the electrodes are positioned too low and therefore pressed against the bed, this may result in artefacts such as in the present example. When this full-term infant with continuous aEEG background was turned (at arrows), a drift in the amplitude of the tracing occurred

Effect of a subgaleal hemorrhage on aEEG amplitude

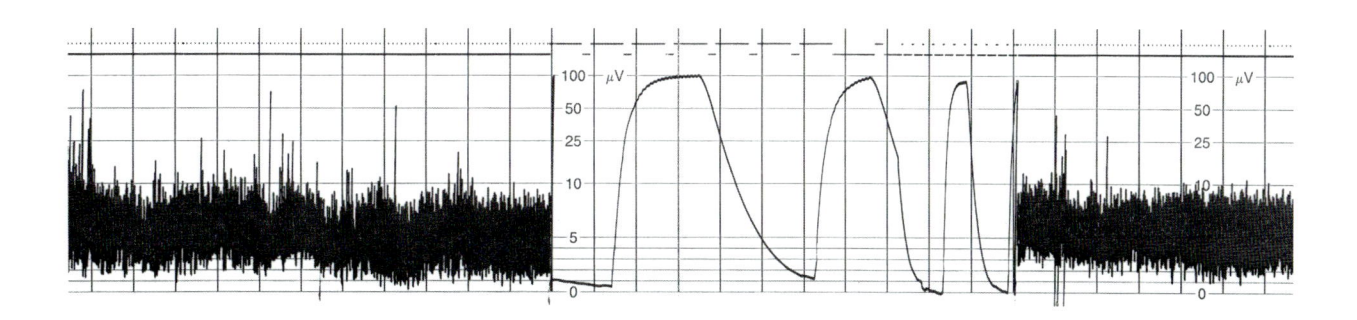

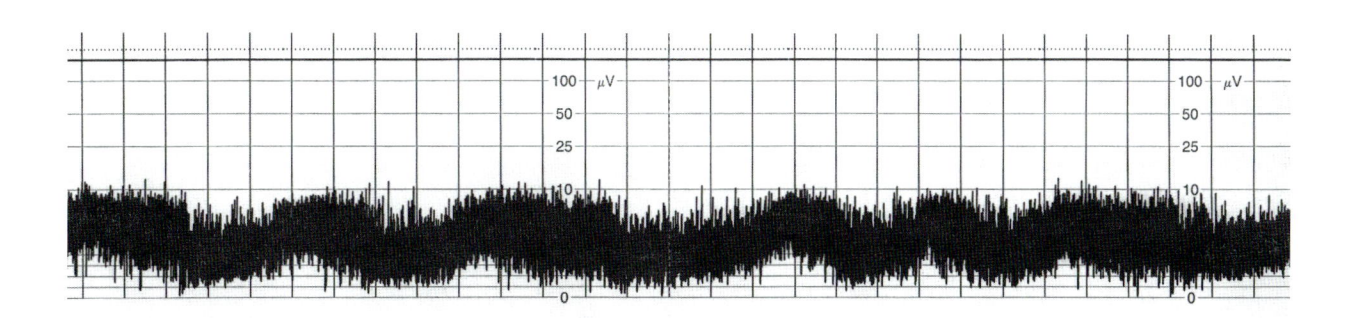

Figure 3.4 This full-term infant was born at 42 weeks' gestation, following the fifth ventouse extraction. He went to the postnatal ward with his mother and fed well to start with, but was found pale, cyanosed and hypothermic in his cot at 8 h of age. His pH was 6.9, the base excess was −24 mmol/l, and the hemoglobin was 4.8 mmol/l. He was noted to have a diffuse subcutaneous swelling consistent with a large subgaleal hemorrhage. He required ventilation and was transferred to the NICU.

The aEEG recording at 20 h shows the effect on aEEG amplitude when the recorded electrocortical activity is dampened by extracranial fluid. As can be seen in the middle of the upper tracing, the level of the amplitude was not due to faulty calibration. The aEEG shows a continuous pattern with cyclical variability suggestive of sleep–wake cycling. He had a normal neurodevelopmental outcome

Effect of a loose electrode

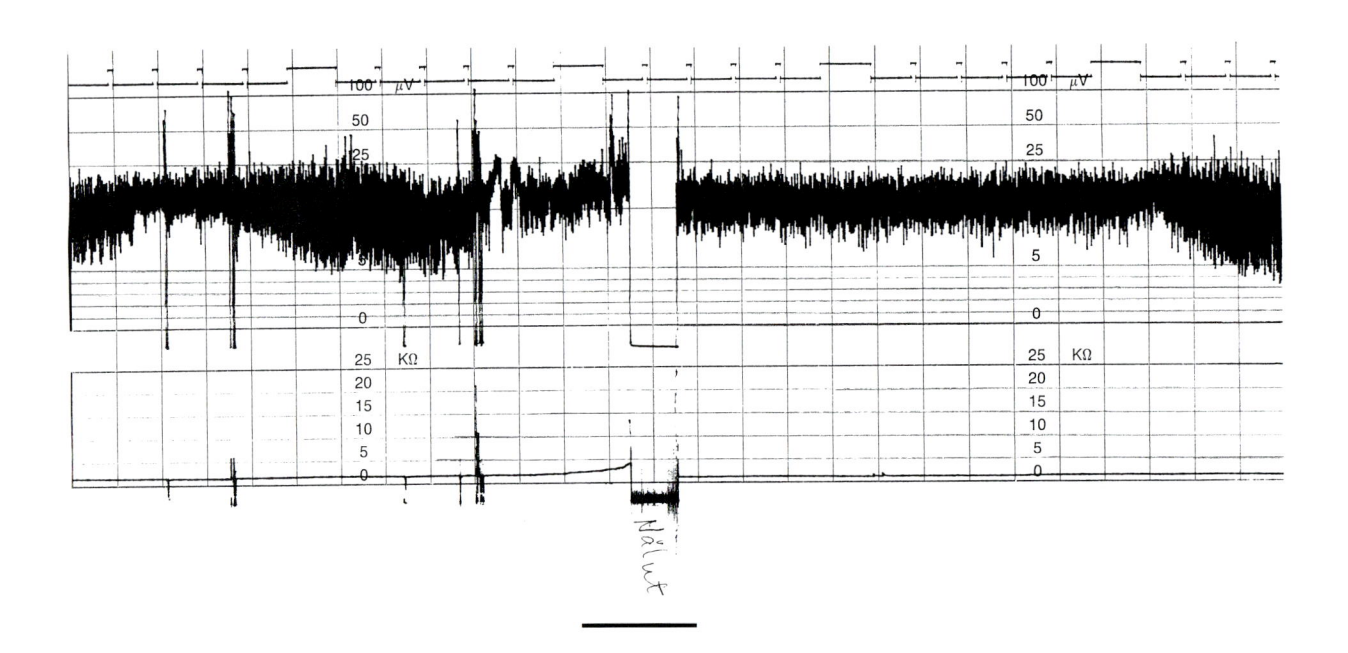

Figure 3.5   This full-term infant had a CNV aEEG with sleep–wake cycling; parts of three quiet-sleep periods can be seen as smooth changes in the minimum aEEG amplitude. In the middle of the recording one electrode came loose and resulted in an interrupted recording. In the CFM, the overload alarm will be alerted and the recording temporarily shut out. The impedance (lower part of the recording) was stable and low, around 2 kΩ, but increased gradually to 5 kΩ during the 10–15 min preceding the time when the electrode went entirely loose. After reattachment of the electrode the tracing proceeded with CNV background and low-electrode impedance

Baseline drift

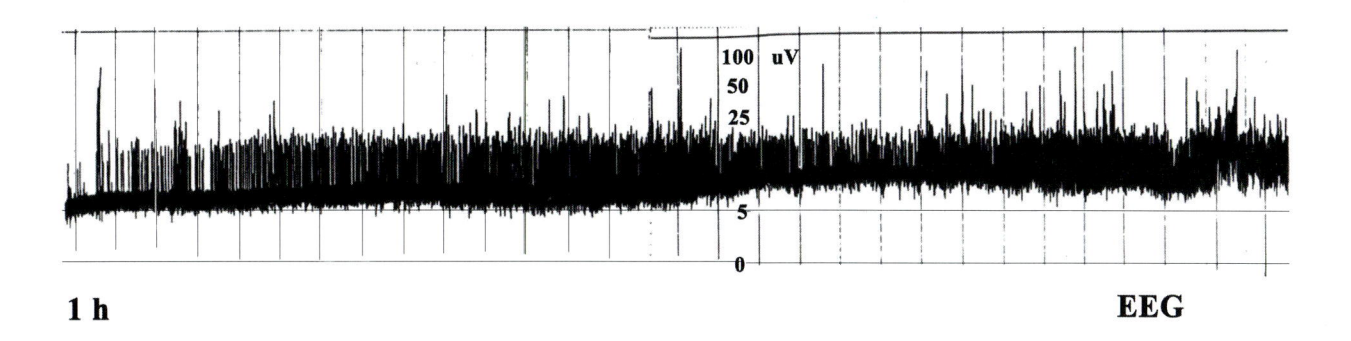

1 h   **EEG**

Figure 3.6   This female infant was born at 40 weeks' gestation following an emergency Cesarean section due to placental abruption. She was immediately intubated and resuscitated. Apgar scores were 2, 5 and 8 at 1, 5 and 10 min, respectively. She developed severe HIE.

The aEEG was calibrated prior to the recording and the impedance was normal. The initial aEEG, recorded from the age of 1 h, showed a low-voltage burst-suppression pattern with a baseline on the 4–5 μV level. The aEEG background recovered with increased burst density during the following hours. A further increase of the aEEG baseline (minimum amplitude) from 5 to 7 μV is difficult to explain but could be due to interference from extracranial activity. The impedance was low, below 5 kΩ (not shown). This drift of the baseline is sometimes seen, especially in infants with severely depressed electrocortical background. It makes interpretation of the trace difficult, as especially the second half could be misinterpreted as CNV. The consequence could be that a child with a severely abnormal trace would not meet the entry criteria used at present for certain intervention trials. The EEG, performed simultaneously, showed a burst-suppression pattern

Background asymmetry due to middle cerebral artery infarction

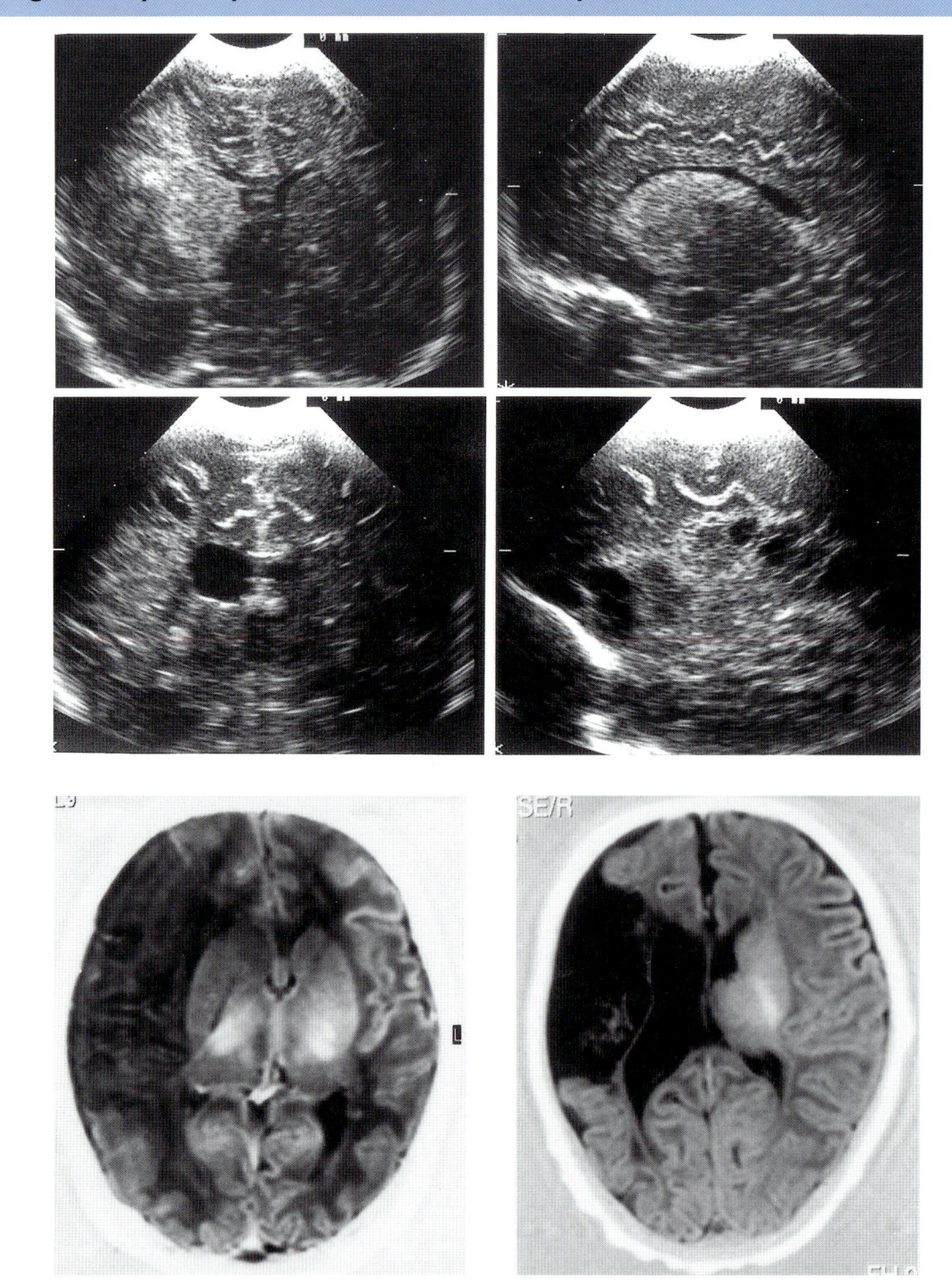

Figure 3.7   This female infant was born at 40 weeks' gestation. The mother had felt decreased fetal movements from about 4 days before the delivery. On arrival at the hospital there was meconium-stained amniotic fluid and decelerations on the cardiotocography. An emergency Cesarean section was performed. The infant was suctioned and bagged briefly, the Apgar scores were 4 at 1 min and 6 at 5 min. At the age of 36 h she had apneic spells and was transferred to the tertiary-level NICU. She had a very abnormal movement pattern with rowing of both arms and legs. She required mechanical ventilation for a few days.

Ultrasound (a) and MRI (b) showed a large right-sided infarction in the distribution of the middle cerebral artery. The infant developed moderate hemiplegia but was able to walk unaided at 18 months of age. She has behavioral problems and mild global delay

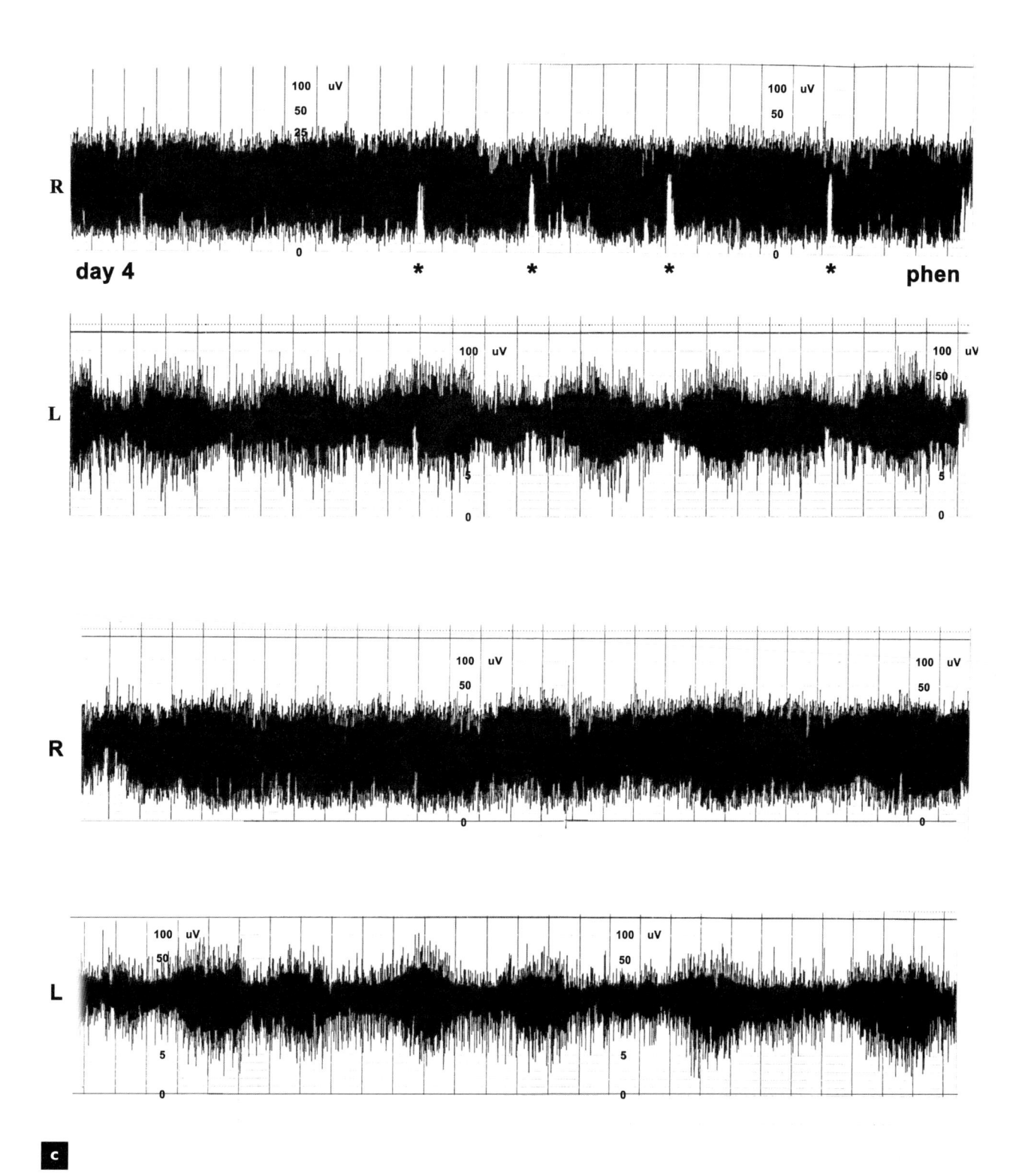

Figure 3.7 continued (c) A bilateral aEEG recording was obtained and showed marked asymmetry in the background activity between the two hemispheres. On the affected right side, the background was discontinuous. On the left side the background was continuous with normal voltage. Sleep–wake cycling is clearly present on the left side but can only be seen on the right side as some variability of the background. Seizures can only be clearly recognized on the right side and appear to respond to administration of phenytoin (phen).

This case is a good example of the potential use of bilateral aEEG recordings in infants with unilateral lesions. Preservation of the electrocortical background of the unaffected hemisphere can be assessed

47

Asymmetry due to hemorrhagic infarction of the posterior cerebral artery

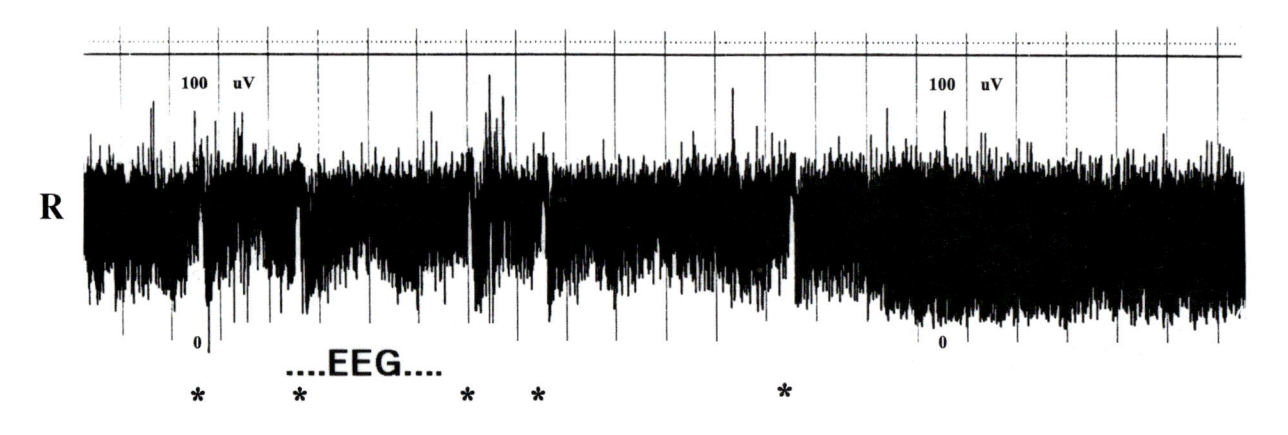

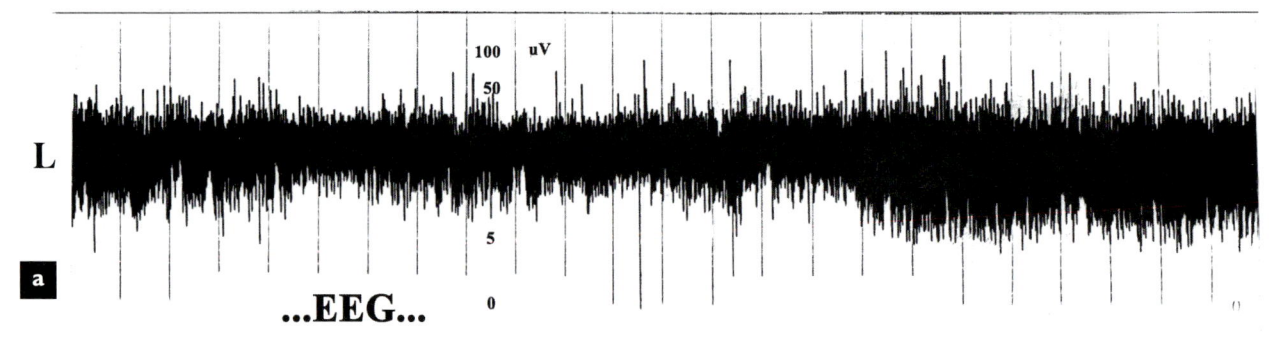

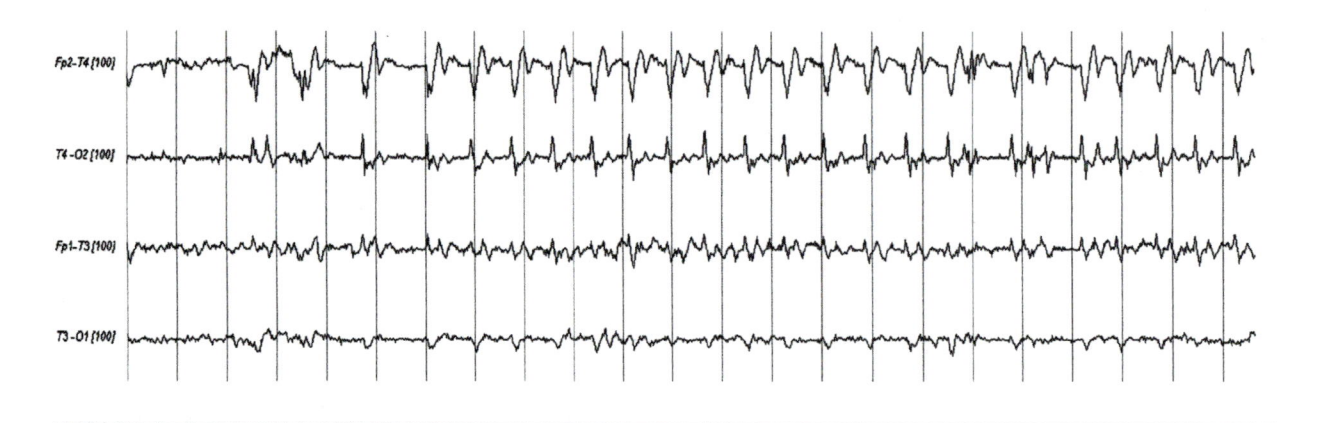

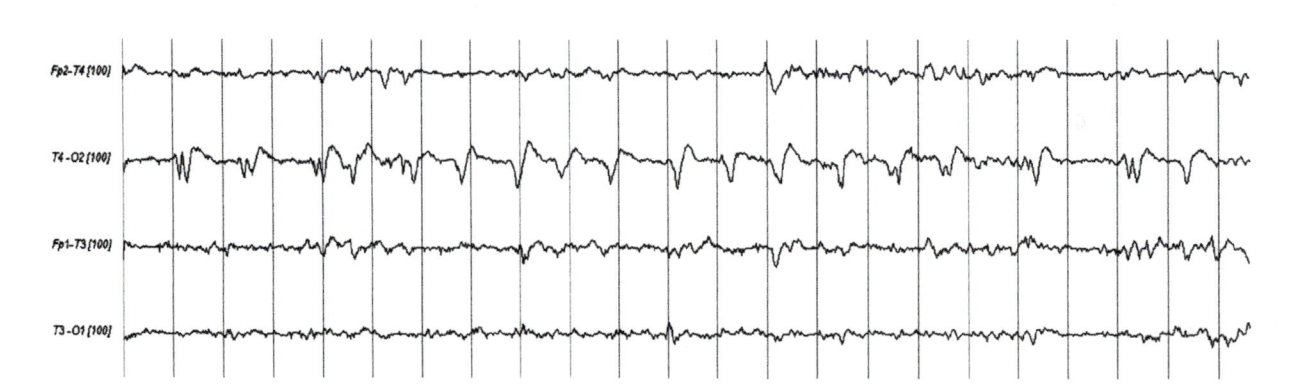

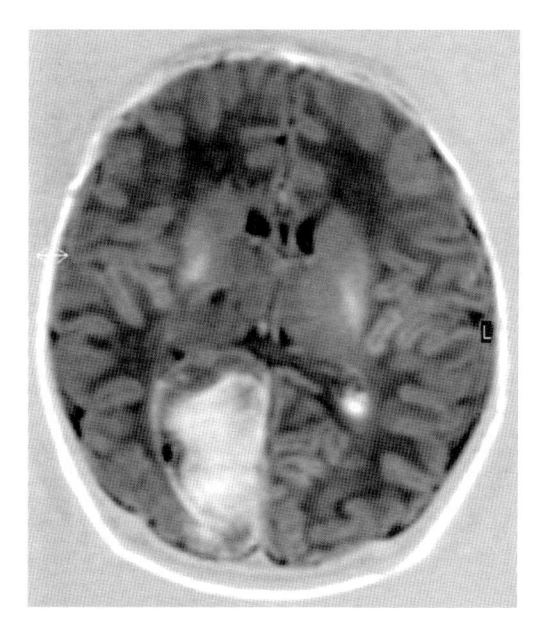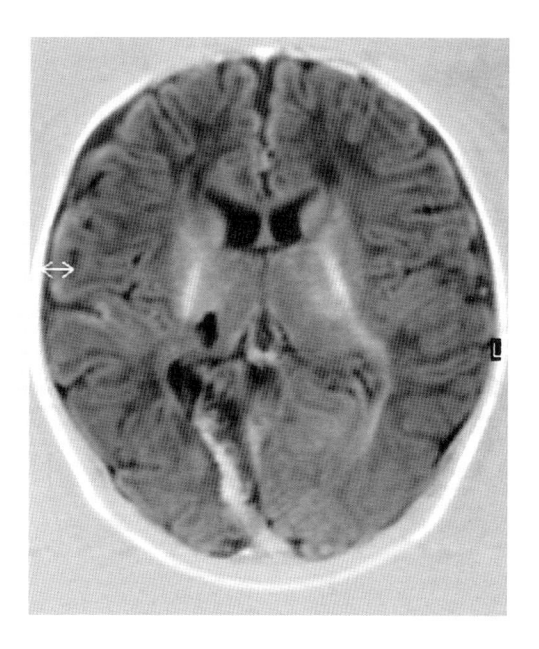

c

Figure 3.8 *opposite and above* This female infant was born at 40 weeks' gestation, following an uncomplicated home delivery. The birth weight was 3500 g, and Apgar scores were 9 and 10 at 1 and 5 min, respectively. Four hours after the delivery she developed hiccups and cyanotic spells, for which she required mechanical ventilation. She also developed focal seizures affecting the left leg.

An ultrasound scan was carried out on admission and MRI was performed on day 6 and again at 3 months. Both examinations showed a right-sided hemorrhagic infarction in the distribution of the posterior cerebral artery, with involvement of the right thalamus. No underlying coagulopathy was detected. Her neurodevelopmental outcome was normal at 2 years.

(a) Since the clinical seizures were focal, and the ultrasound showed a unilateral lesion, a two-channel aEEG recording was obtained. The simultaneous aEEG from the two hemispheres showed clear asymmetry, with a slightly depressed but continuous background on the right side (R) and a continuous normal voltage background on the left side (L). The epileptic seizure activity was dominating on the right side (asterisks). The epileptic seizure activity can also be identified on the left side although it is not as obvious as on the right side. Reproduced from reference 44 with permission (*Pediatrics* vol. 109, pages 772–9, Figure 1, Copyright 2002).

(b) Simultaneously with the aEEG, a standard EEG was recorded. The upper EEG trace shows focal repetitive sharp waves over the right temporal region (T4). However, another focal seizure arising in the right occipital lobe (lower EEG trace) was not recognized in the aEEG. Following administration of midazolam, the electrographic seizure activity was interrupted and the background became more depressed on both sides. Reproduced from reference 44 with permission (*Pediatrics* vol. 109, pages 772–9, Figure 1, Copyright 2002).

This example shows that, in infants with unilateral lesions, a bilateral recording with two channels gives additional information.

(c) MRI using inversion recovery sequence, performed in the neonatal period (left) and at 3 months (right) showing a hemorrhagic infarction in the region of the posterior cerebral artery

4

aEEG and neonatal seizures

Detection of epileptic seizure activity is one of the main indications for aEEG monitoring in newborn infants. Epileptic seizures are relatively common in ill and distressed newborn infants. The seizures are often reactive and caused by transient disturbances in cerebral oxygenation, metabolism and blood flow. The most common etiologies to neonatal seizures include hypoxia–ischemia, intracranial hemorrhages, metabolic disturbance (e.g. hypoglycemia) and intracranial infections. Congenital cerebral malformations are relatively rare but may cause severe and recurrent seizures.

The incidence of neonatal seizures in a NICU population is dependent on the patient population, the diagnostic criteria and the diagnostic methods[54–56]. When epileptic seizure activity in a standard EEG recording was a criterion for neonatal seizure diagnosis, the incidence in a NICU population was 2.3%[57]. When standard EEG and aEEG were combined to diagnose infants with seizures, we obtained an incidence of 4.5% of neonatal seizures in our NICU[56]. However, the prevalence of epileptic seizure activity may be as high as 20% when continuous EEG monitoring is used in selected high-risk populations[58,59]. Electrographic seizures are probably not uncommon in infants during extracorporeal membrane oxygenation (ECMO)[60]. Up to 65–75% of preterm infants developing germinal matrix hemorrhages (GMH–IVH) or other hemorrhagic–ischemic lesions have epileptic seizure activity, often subtle or entirely subclinical[39,61–63]. Moderately preterm infants (30–36 weeks' gestation) seem to have the lowest incidence of seizures[64].

There are some features of newborn epileptic seizures that are specific for the neonatal period:

(1) A majority of neonatal seizures are subclinical or have only subtle clinical symptoms[65,66]. It is not uncommon that NICU patients have subclinical seizures lasting for several hours[67–70]. It is also not uncommon that clinical epileptic seizures continue as subclinical epileptic seizures when antiepileptic medications are administered[9,56,58,71].

(2) Neonatal clinical seizures can be difficult to distinguish from other movements. Mizrahi and Kellaway[72] used EEG video monitoring and showed that clinically suspected seizures often do not have corresponding electrographic seizure activity. A method for distinguishing clinical epileptic seizures from other movements has been suggested by Volpe[73]. Jittery movements, sleep myoclonus and other non-epileptic phenomena often cease if slight restraint is put on the moving limb, e.g. by the observer's hand, while movements elicited by epileptic seizure activity continues.

(3) Most newborn infants with seizures have both clinical and subclinical seizures. The aEEG samples in this chapter show examples of the various behaviors of neonatal seizures.

(4) Neonatal seizures are difficult to diagnose by clinical observation only. A diagnostic approach including close clinical observation or video monitoring, EEG monitoring of high-risk infants and standard EEG is optimal in order to diagnose neonatal seizures correctly.

Neonatal seizures are associated with increased mortality and adverse neurological outcome[54,57,74–77]. Intractable seizures and seizures associated with severely abnormal EEG background have the worst prognosis[55,78–82]. Recent data indicate that subclinical seizures and brief rhythmic discharges are also associated with poor outcome[83,84]. Seizures are not associated with poor outcome in asphyxiated infants with HIE, but are correlated with worse outcome in infants with moderate to severe HIE[85]. Treatment of subclinical seizure activity may be associated with lower risk for later recurrence, although this has not been investigated in randomized controlled studies[56]. Studies investigating possible adverse effects on the newborn brain from seizure activity give different results[86–91]. There are different views on whether subclinical seizures need treatment or not, but it is outside the scope of this Atlas to discuss subclinical seizures further. However, it seems reasonable to conclude that it is important to diagnose subclinical epileptic seizure activity in newborn infants in order for the neonatologist to make appropriate decisions.

Epileptic seizures have varying clinical and electrographic characteristics. Epileptic seizures may be focal or generalized. The seizures may appear single or as repetitive seizures with variable durations and variable interseizure intervals. The electrographic components or complexes are usually rhythmic and vary in frequency, amplitude, duration and localization. The minimum duration for a rhythmic EEG pattern to be classified as a neonatal seizure varies between different studies, but is usually at least 5–10 s. Two review articles on definitions and problems with classification of neonatal seizures are recommended[82,92]. Neonatal EEG seizure patterns are sometimes difficult to diagnose since they may be continuously ongoing, of very low voltage and they do not always contain sharp-wave activity. Figure 4.1 is an example of an aEEG and an EEG where the seizure pattern was actually easier to identify in the aEEG than in the EEG.

(1) Epileptic seizure activity in the aEEG is discernible because it represents a transitory change (in both frequency and amplitude) of the electrocortical background activity.

(2) Epileptic seizure activity in the aEEG is usually characterized by a transient rise in the background activity. The most common finding is a rapid rise of both the lower and the upper margins of the tracing (see the examples below). Recurrent epileptic seizure activity in the aEEG, corresponding to status epilepticus or serial seizures, looks like a 'saw-tooth' (Figures 4.1, 4.2 and 4.3).

(3) The desynchronization of the EEG in hypsarrhythmia during infantile spasms results in a transient decrease of the aEEG amplitude (Figure 4.4).

Neonatal seizures may be misdiagnosed in the aEEG for the following reasons:

(1) Brief seizure activity can be difficult to diagnose, as can be seen in Figure 4.5c. It may not be possible to detect very brief seizure activity with the aEEG[42,44].

(2) If the epileptic seizure activity is continuous without interruption, there is a risk that it may be overlooked since there is no change of the aEEG background amplitude (Figure 4.6). This is relatively rare, but should be suspected in aEEG recordings with continuous very high amplitude. A standard EEG reveals the seizure activity.

(3) Arousal during care procedures often results in a transient rise of the aEEG background and may be misinterpreted as epileptic seizure activity. It is important that all care procedures are documented on the tracing to facilitate correct interpretation.

(4) The limited number of electrodes makes the aEEG method easy to use for clinical routine monitoring. However, one must be aware that some very focal epileptic seizure activity may also be missed (Figure 3.8)[42,44].

- The aEEG increases the possibilities of detecting neonatal epileptic seizure activity;

- The aEEG should be used as a complement to standard EEG;

- The aEEG is very useful for monitoring responses to anticonvulsive treatment;

- Since the cerebral function monitor (CFM) does not provide raw EEG there is a certain risk for over- and underinterpretation of epileptic seizure activity. Newer techniques for aEEG monitoring, with possibilities of inspecting the raw EEG, will reduce these risks (see Figures 1.7 and 1.9).

aEEG and EEG seizure patterns

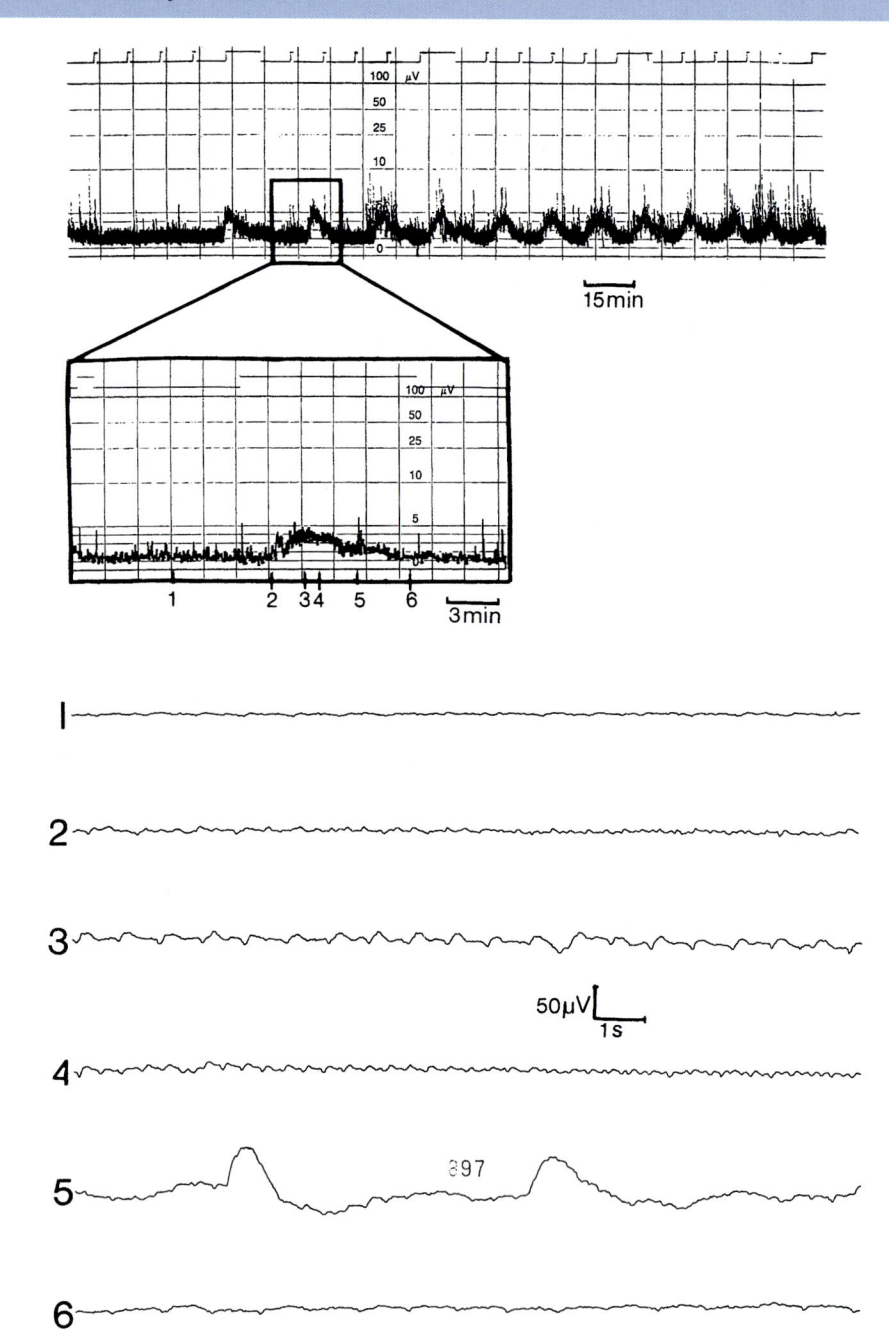

Figure 4.1   Simultaneous recording of an EEG and aEEG in a severely asphyxiated full-term infant with subclinical seizures who died due to the severe brain injury. The duration of the aEEG tracing is almost 4 h.

(a) The aEEG is characterized by a low voltage 'saw-tooth' pattern consisting of recurrent low-amplitude epileptic seizure activity superimposed on an extremely low-voltage, mainly inactive, background.

(b) The numbers before the raw EEG tracings (1–6) correspond with the numbers in the aEEG during a selected 20-min period. The raw EEG tracings show a gradual build-up and decrease of repetitive low-voltage sharp-wave activity. In EEG tracing number 5, two movement artefacts are present; they are also discernible in the aEEG tracing. The epileptic seizure activity was entirely subclinical. Reproduced from reference 42 with permission.

This example shows the correspondence between seizure patterns in aEEG and EEG. The extremely low-voltage electro-cortical background activity is predictive of very poor outcome

aEEG seizure patterns

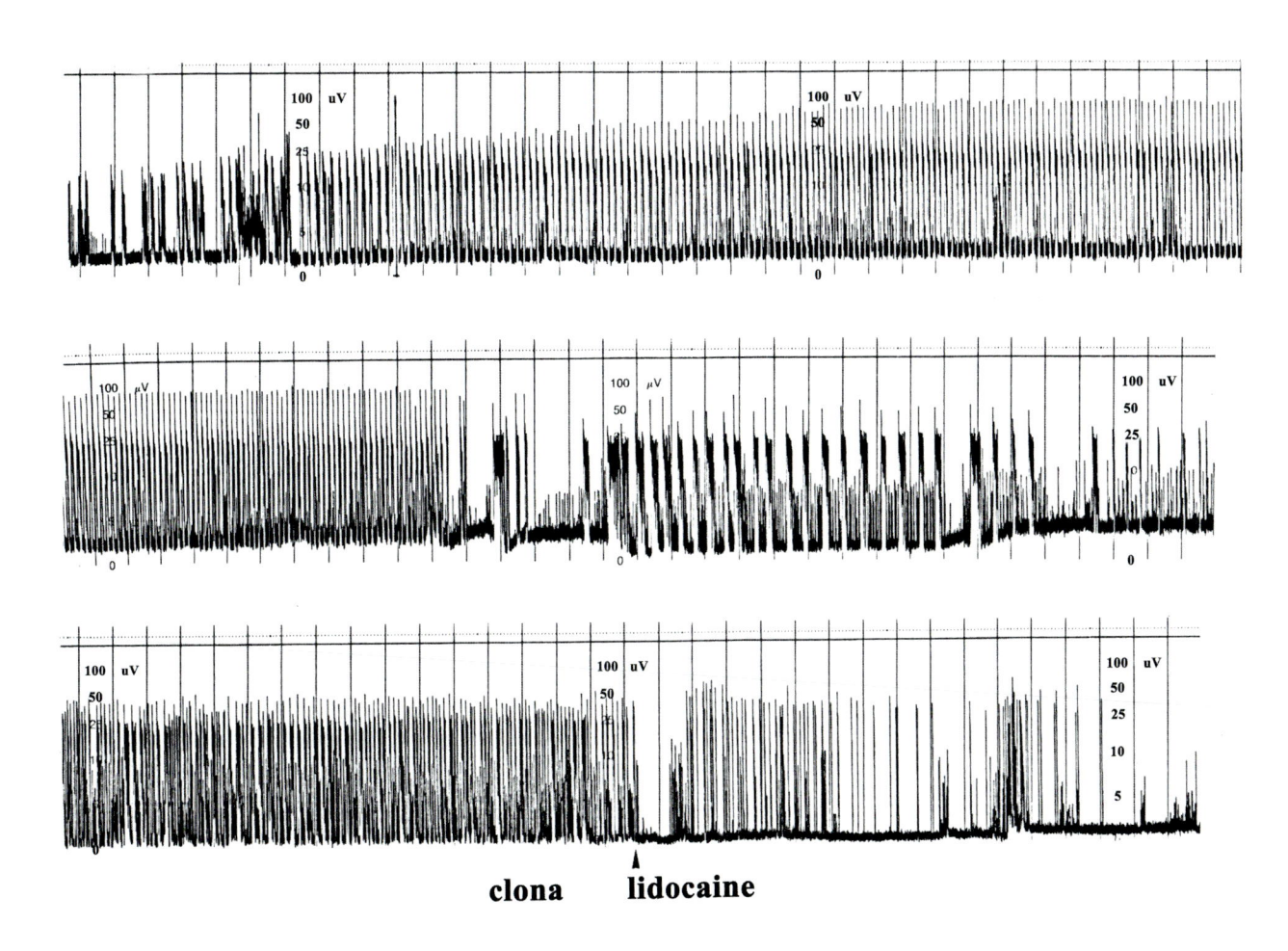

clona   lidocaine

Figure 4.2   This full-term female infant suffered severe perinatal asphyxia, following a ruptured uterus. The aEEG recording was started in the evening and continued overnight. As the CFM was still new and the experience limited, the status epilepticus that was present all night long was not recognized. The child did not show any obvious clinical seizures, but the ventilatory support was changed from endotracheal continuous positive airway pressure (CPAP) to ventilation, because of lack of ventilatory drive.

The top aEEG trace can easily be mistaken for a burst-suppression pattern, but when looking more closely the baseline is repetitively interrupted. In the middle part of the recording the seizure discharges become more 'typical', with longer duration of individual seizures, and are therefore easier to recognize. When the status epilepticus in the aEEG was recognized, clonazepam (clona) was administered without any success. Lidocaine was subsequently administered and this drug was effective in stopping the electrographic seizures. This 'saw-tooth' pattern, with repetitive seizures on a mainly inactive background, is predictive of poor outcome

aEEG seizure patterns – inactivity and sudden electrographic seizures

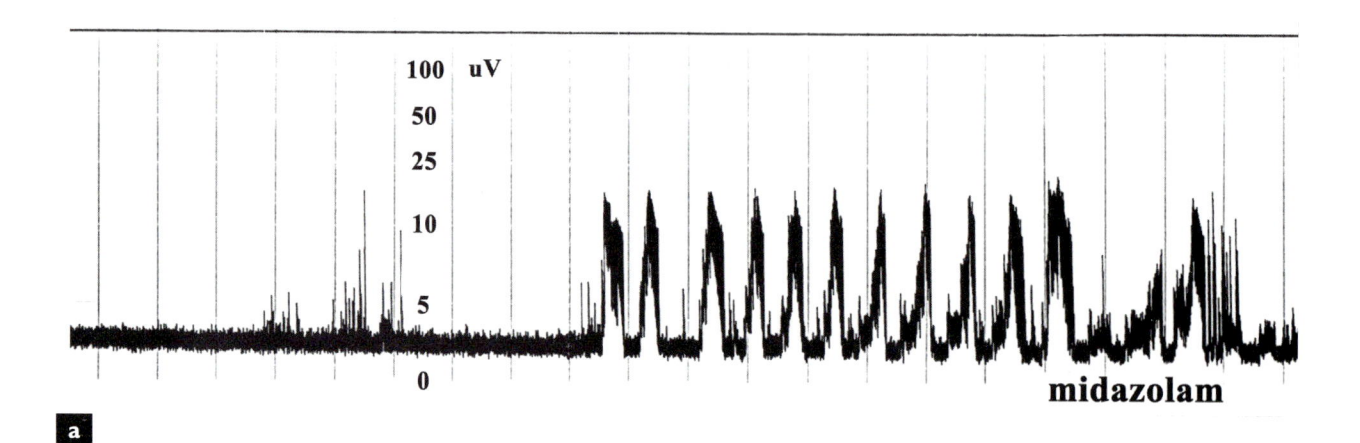

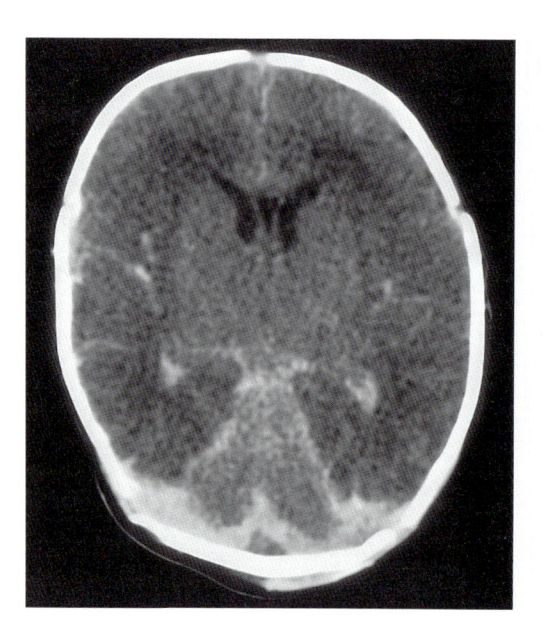
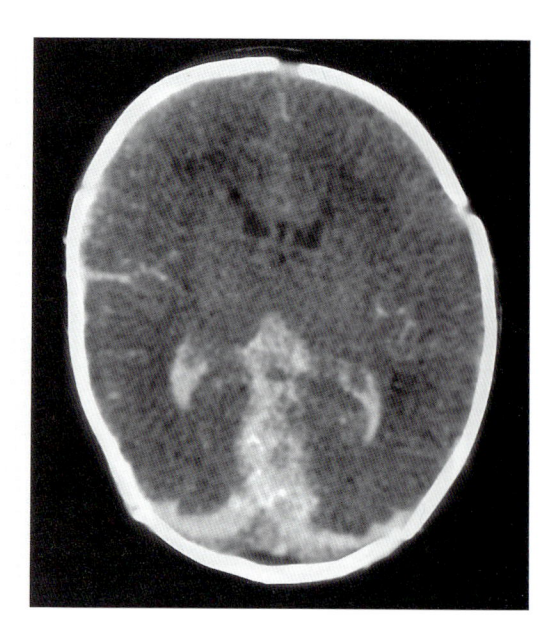

Figure 4.3   This male infant was born at 40 weeks' gestation by a difficult vaginal breech delivery. His Apgar scores were 4 and 6 at 1 and 5 min, respectively. His birth weight was 3200 g. At 8 h he deteriorated with clinical seizures and needed resuscitation. Following stabilization he was transferred to the NICU. The first arterial pH was 6.80 with a base excess of –27 mmol/l and an arterial lactate level of 24 mmol/l.

A large hemorrhage in the posterior fossa, also involving the cerebellum, was suspected on ultrasound and confirmed on computerized tomography (CT). Fractures of the skull at the level of the sella turcica and at the border of the parietal and occipital bone were also present. He was flaccid and had no spontaneous respiration, and died. The postmortem examination showed extensive neuronal loss in the hippocampus, layer III and V of the cortex, in the thalami and basal ganglia as well as the large hemorrhages in the posterior fossa and the cerebellum. A tentorial tear was also present.

(a) Following admission to the NICU at 10 h of age, the aEEG was started and showed an entirely flat background. This finding was confirmed by standard EEG. Several hours later, a sudden electrographic status epilepticus appeared in the aEEG. The duration of each seizure was around 5 min with a flat interictal period also lasting around 5 min. Midazolam was administered and resulted in a somewhat lower amplitude of the seizure activity and slightly increased interictal duration.

(b) A CT scan performed on day 1 showed a large subdural collection in the posterior fossa as well as an intraventricular hemorrhage and loss of grey–white matter differentiation throughout both hemispheres.

This type of recording is unusual, with an inactive background abruptly changing into an electrographic status epilepticus

aEEG seizure patterns with downward deflection

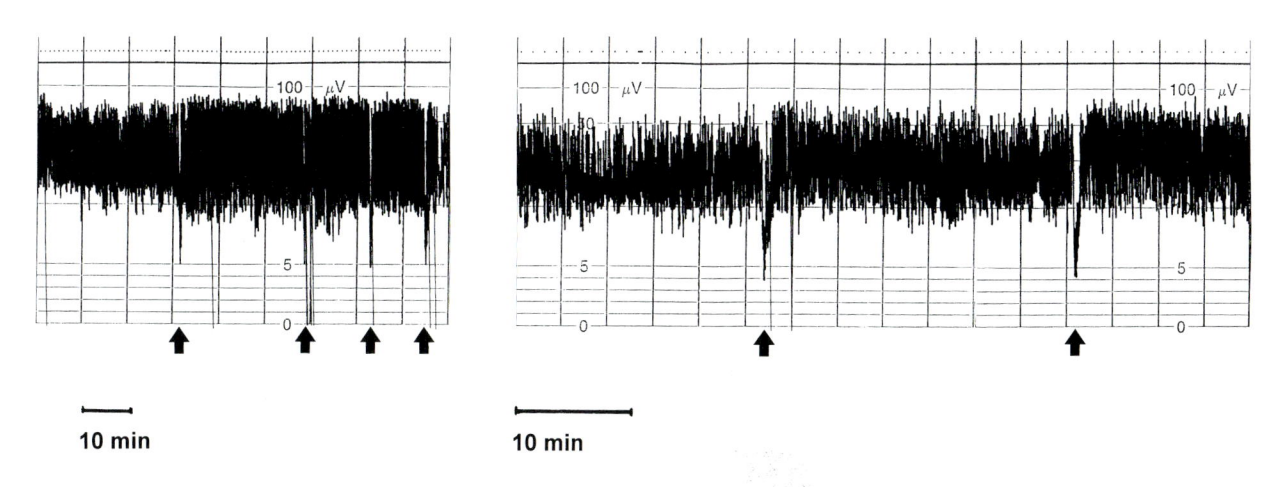

10 min   10 min

a

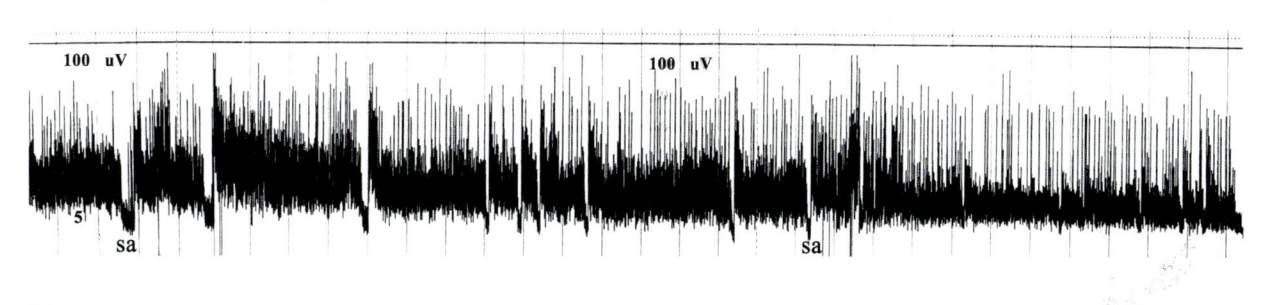

b

Figure 4.4   (a) The pregnancy and delivery of this 2-month-old male infant was normal, and he was initially doing well. However, at the age of 2 months he developed infantile spasms and the EEG showed hypsarrhythmia. The left aEEG shows four very short, abrupt decreases in amplitude that occurred simultaneously with clinical seizures and corresponded to a generalized attenuation of EEG activity, which is usually seen during infantile spasms. The deflections are easier to see in the aEEG tracing on the right recorded with faster paper speed (30 cm/h). The EEG from this infant showed multifocal interictal epileptiform activity, and a typical desynchronization episode. In the trend analysis of the total power recorded from one EEG channel (C3) this seizure coinicided with a sharp drop in power.

(b) This example shows a full-term infant with HIE. The seizure pattern in the aEEG is similar to the hypsarrythmic aEEG seen in (a). The brief periods with downward deflections on a burst-suppression background were associated with drops in the infant's saturation (sa)

Seizure patterns that may be difficult to diagnose with the aEEG

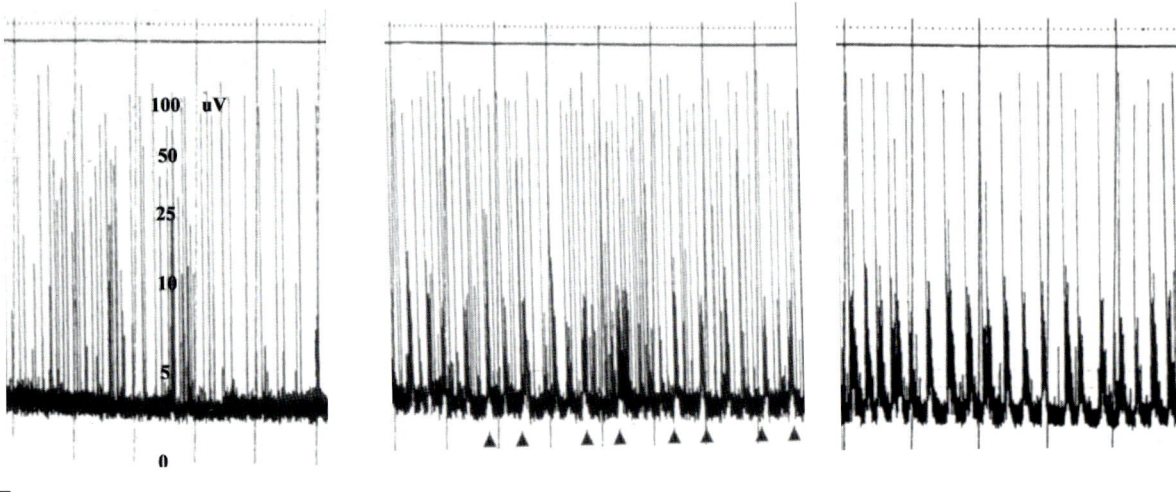

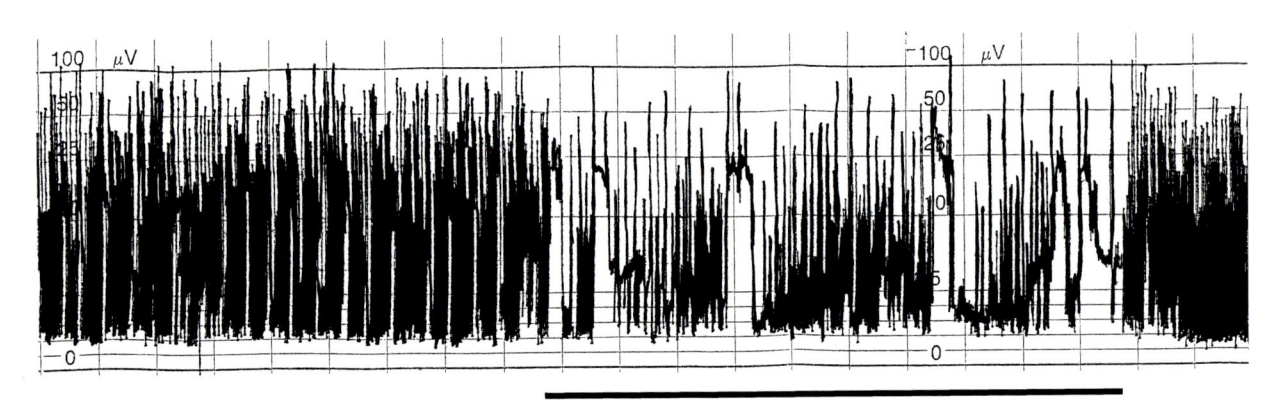

Figure 4.5   (a) These three short examples show the difference between a burst-suppression background pattern with relatively low burst density (left), and two seizure patterns (middle and right). The background is severely depressed in all three tracings. The middle and right tracings, with seizure patterns, are characterized by the interrupted baselines that occur with 2–5-min intervals and with a duration of 1–2 min.

(b) Short repetitive seizures on a discontinuous background. The burst-suppression background in this example is characterized by a relatively high burst density and repeated short interruptions in the minimum amplitude. The suspected seizure pattern was more evident when the paper speed was changed from 6 cm/h to 30 cm/h (underlined)

Single seizures with a short duration

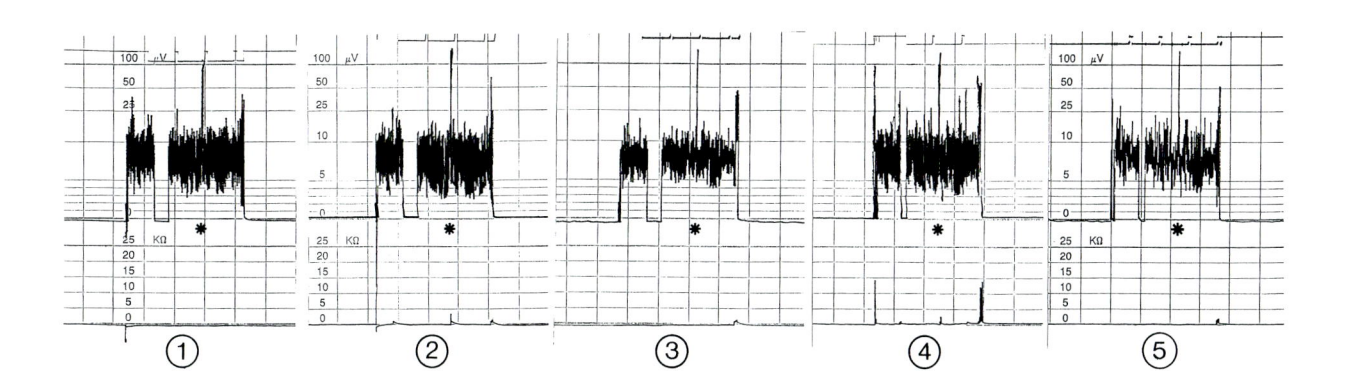

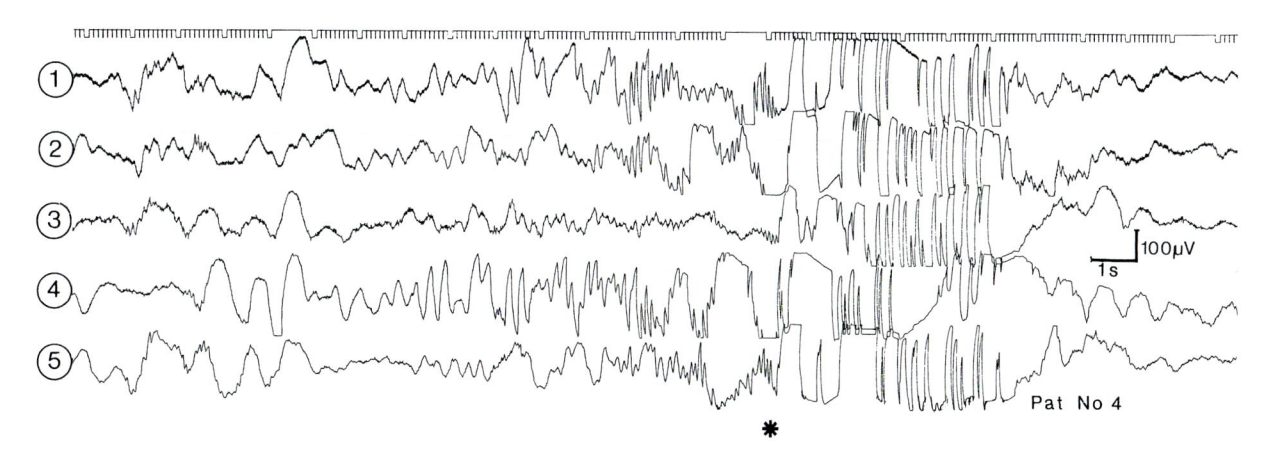

100μV

1s

Pat No 4

c

Figure 4.5 continued (c) This short recording shows five channels of simultaneously recorded EEG and aEEG. Channels 1 and 2 were recorded from the left hemisphere (Fp1–C3 and C3–P3), and channels 3 and 4 from the right hemisphere (Fp2–C4, C4–P4). Channel 5 was the standard biparietal electrode (P3–P4) in aEEG recordings. The electrocortical background is continuous. The recording was first interrupted for 5 min due to a loose electrode. Shortly thereafter a short generalized seizure, lasting only 10 s, occurred. The seizure can be seen in all five aEEG tracings as a short burst of high-amplitude activity (marked with an asterisk), clearly different from the continuous background activity. It is too short to cause a shift in basline, and is difficult to discriminate from an artefact. Reproduced from reference 42 with permission

Seizure patterns that may be difficult to diagnose with the aEEG

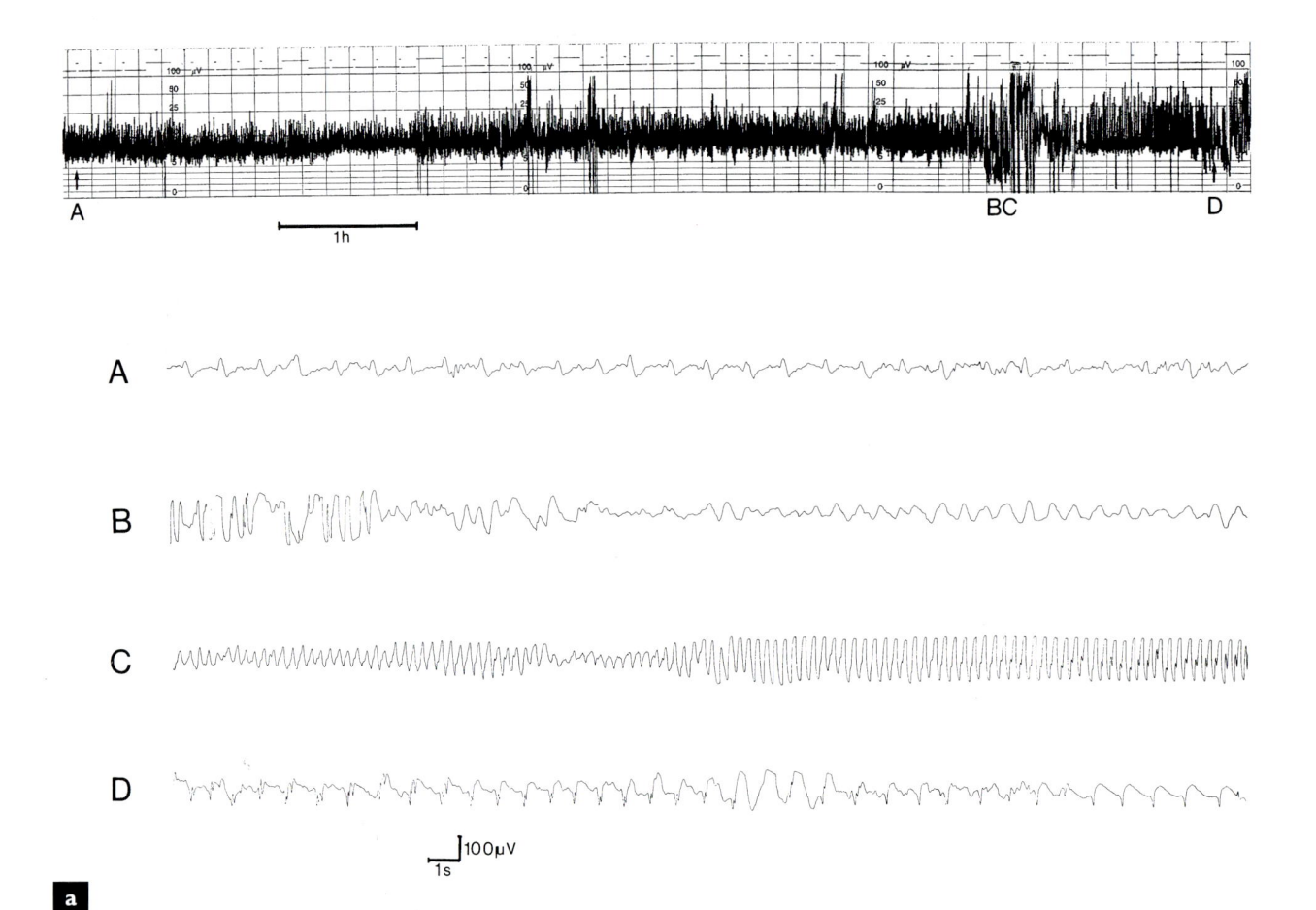

Figure 4.6 *above and opposite* Continuous seizure activity. This full-term male infant was initially doing well, but on the second day of life he developed clinical seizures. Clinical investigations showed that he had a metabolic disorder, ornithine-transcarbamylase deficiency, from which he also died in spite of intensive care treatment.

(a) The aEEG was started with a simultaneous recording of the raw EEG on a Medilog EEG tape recorder. At 'A' the raw EEG revealed 20 min of continuously ongoing seizure activity that was not possible to detect in the aEEG. The infant did not have any clinical seizures at this time. At 'B' and 'C' he developed severe apneic spells; the EEG but not the aEEG showed high-voltage seizure activity. After 'C' there are some movement artefacts corresponding to the infant being intubated. At 'D' new seizure activity recurred and can also be seen in the aEEG.

(b) The second aEEG tracing from this infant showed a very high-amplitude 'saw-tooth' pattern (E to G) that corresponded to almost continuous seizure activity in the EEG. The epileptic seizure activity in the EEG also continued at 'H' and 'I', but is not so obvious in the aEEG although it can be suspected. The aEEG pattern is abnormal, with high-amplitude activity. When tracings like this (H and I) are seen in the aEEG, a standard EEG should be performed in order to rule out epileptic seizure activity. From 'J' to 'L' the aEEG background became increasingly discontinuous. The aEEG diagnosed no further epileptic seizure activity. This infant did not have any clinical seizures from 'E' to 'I', but he was very unstable with recurrent cardiac arrhythmias. Reproduced from reference 42 with permission.

This figure shows that epileptic seizure activity can be overlooked in the aEEG if the epileptic seizure pattern resembles the interictal background activity in amplitude and frequency distribution. Furthermore, very-high-amplitude aEEG patterns may represent continuously ongoing epileptic seizure activity which should be ruled out, or confirmed, by a standard EEG

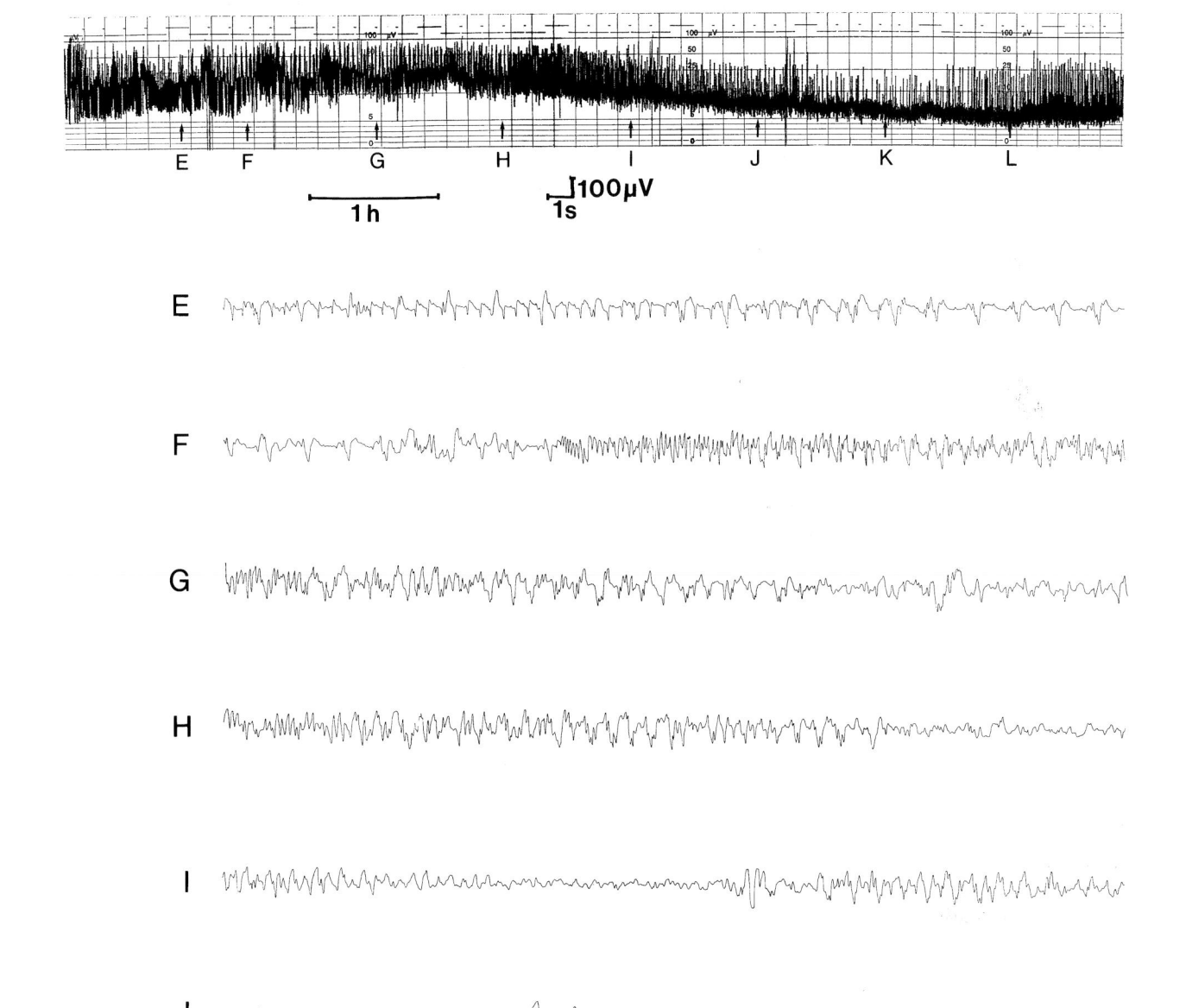

Effects of lidocaine and midazolam on aEEG seizure patterns

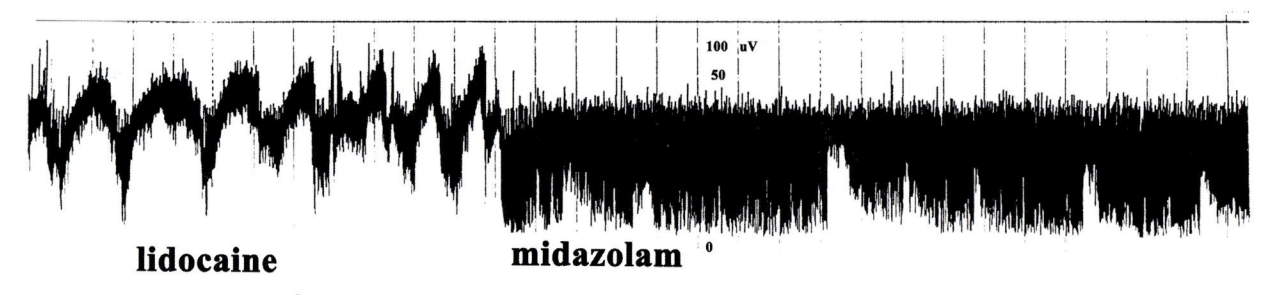

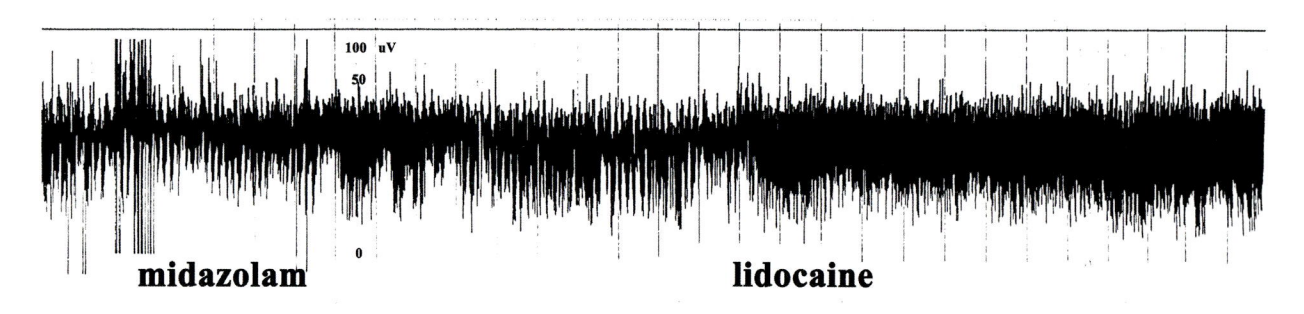

Figure 4.7 The recordings from these two children show that the effect of anticonvulsive therapy is hard to predict and that the drugs administered are not always effective.

(a) The upper aEEG tracing shows a full-term infant with severe perinatal asphyxia, who developed recurrent epileptic seizures and received phenobarbitone before the aEEG recording was initiated. The aEEG shows that when he was given lidocaine there was no apparent effect on the seizures. However, following administration of midazolam the status epilepticus was temporarily interrupted, but seizures recurred a few hours later.

(b) In the second full-term infant, with moderate perinatal asphyxia, midazolam was given following phenobarbitone administration with no apparent effect. Somewhat later the administration of lidocaine does result in a discontinuation of electrographic discharges. Reproduced from reference 53 with permission

Clinical seizures continue as subclinical seizure activity

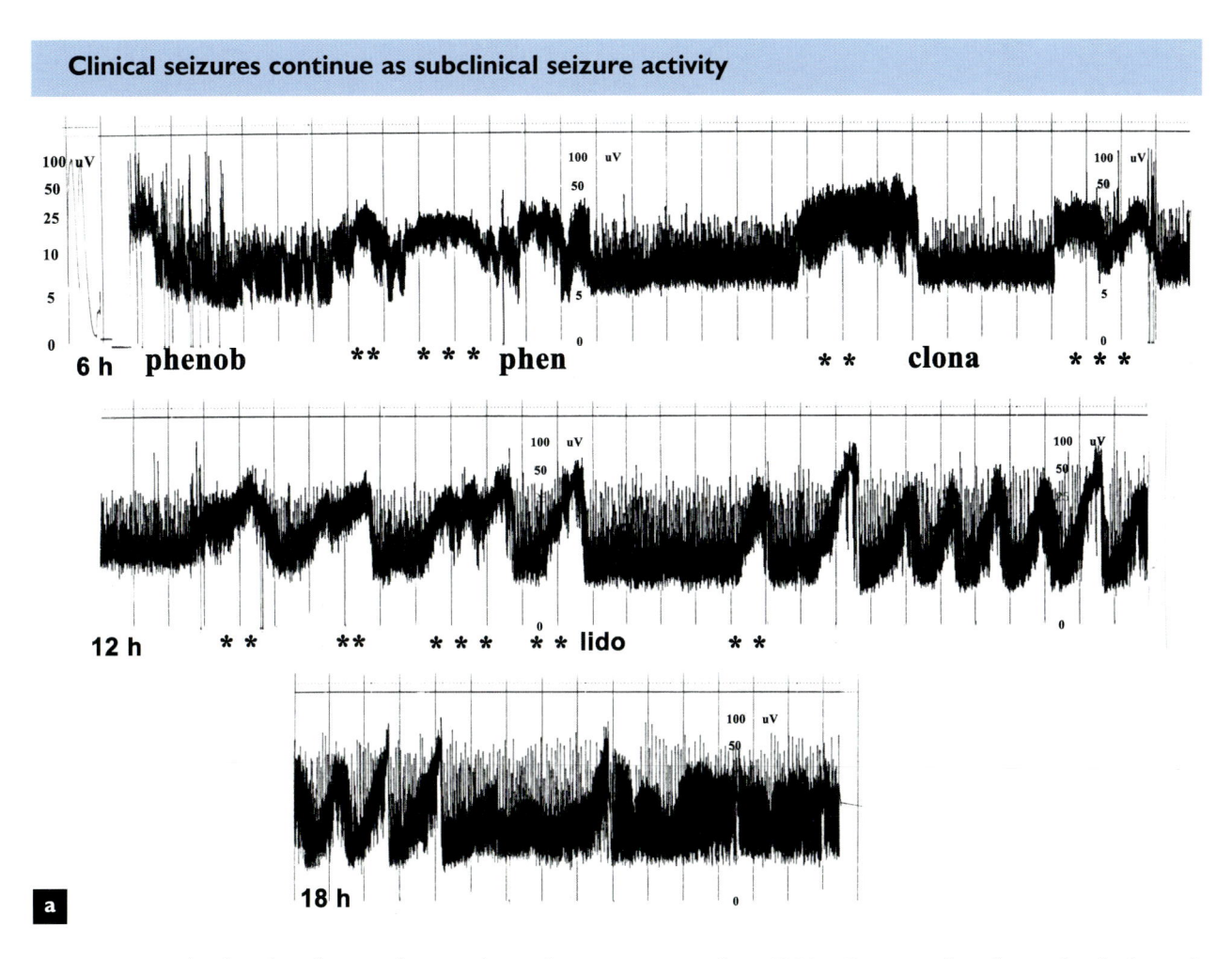

Figure 4.8 This female infant was born at 41 weeks' gestation, weighing 3390 g. For some days the mother had noted decreased fetal movements. During the delivery the CTG showed decreased variability and decelerations, and the amniotic fluid was heavily meconium-stained. The infant was born vaginally with Apgar scores 1, 3 and 5 at 1, 5 and 10 min, respectively. The umbilical arterial pH was 6.75 with a base excess of –24 mmol/l. She was intubated and ventilated for a short period until spontaneous respiration occurred. At 2 h of age the blood glucose was low (1.6 mmol/l) but rose to 2.3 mmol/l 3 h later. Five hours after delivery she started to have clinical seizures for which she was given 0.5 mg of diazepam rectally. She was then intubated and referred to the NICU. On admission she had a pH of 7.34 and a base excess of –5.1 mmol/l and an arterial lactate level of 7.8 mmol/l. She required mild ventilatory support for the first 5 days. She did not require any inotropic support.

Cranial ultrasound and MRI showed severe abnormalities suggestive of parasagittal watershed injury, more marked in the occipital region. Evoked responses revealed an auditory brainstem response only at 90 dB, a delayed visual evoked potential and a consistently normal somatosensory evoked potential (SEP). These findings indicate sensorineural hearing loss, visual perception problems, but probably not development of cerebral palsy since the SEP was consistently normal[93].

At 6 weeks of age subcortical cysts could be seen using ultrasound through the posterior fontanelle. A repeat MRI at 3 months of age showed extensive watershed injury. At 5 years of age, she had become severely microcephalic, with an IQ < 50. She was wearing hearing aids for severe perceptive hearing loss, but had not developed cerebral palsy and she was able to walk unaided.

On admission to the NICU, the aEEG (a) was started immediately. A loading dose of phenobarbitone (phenob; 20 mg/kg intravenously) was given but she went on to have clinical (at asterisks) and subclinical seizures. She was given phenytoin (phen; 15 mg/kg intravenously), followed by clonazepam (clona; 0.1 mg/kg intravenously), and finally a loading dose of lidocaine (lido; 2 mg/kg intravenously) followed by a continuous intravenous infusion (6 mg/kg/h). In spite of all this medication she continued to have repetitive seizures for a prolonged period of time. While her seizures were initially mainly clinical, the latter part of the aEEG recording mainly shows subclinical seizure activity of shorter duration than the previous clinical seizures

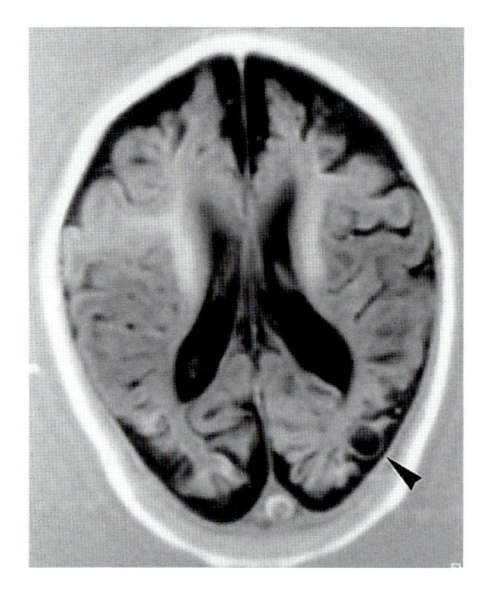

b

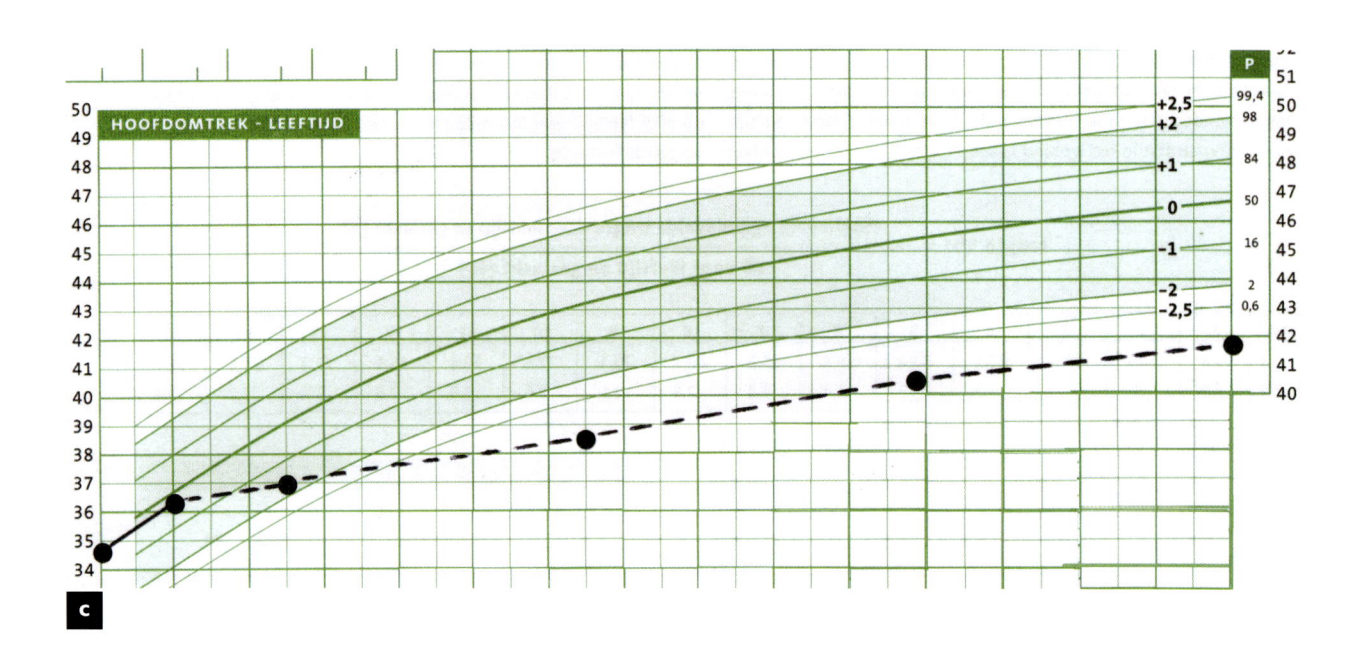

c

Figure 4.8 continued   (b) MRI, using inversion recovery sequence, performed at 3 months of age, shows a pattern sugges-tive of parasagittal watershed injury, with subcortical lesions (arrowhead) and cortical atrophy. Reproduced from reference 94 with permission.

(c) Head circumference, showing a drop from the 50th to below the –2.5 standard deviation centile between birth and 15 months of age

Clinical seizures continue as subclinical seizure activity

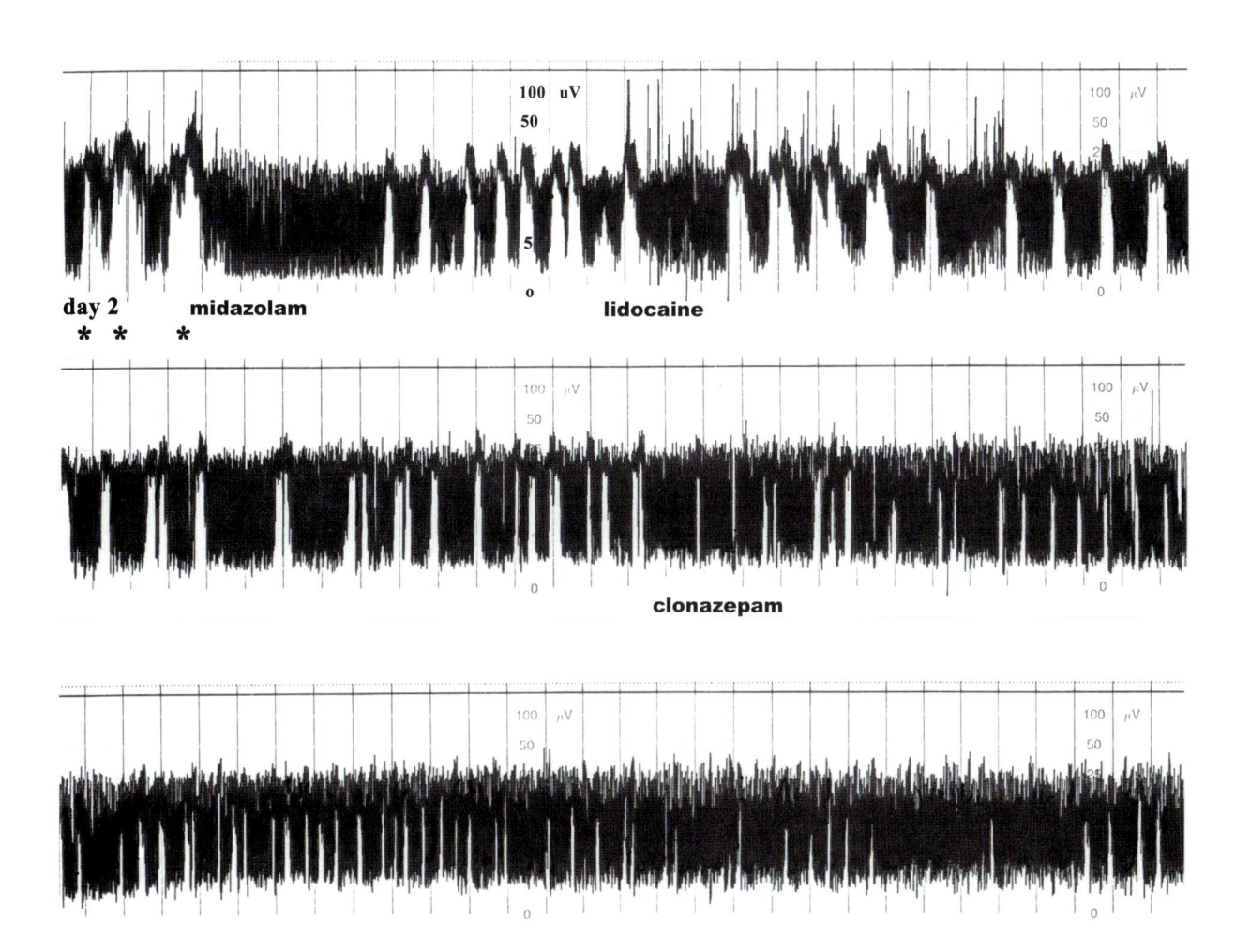

Figure 4.9   This female infant with moderate HIE was born at term, weighing 3450 g. The pregnancy was complicated by hypertension. She was delivered by ventouse extraction and was reported to have a poor start, but Apgar scores were not reported. She was admitted to the neonatal unit and was irritable for a few hours but then started to drink. The next day convulsions were first noted and she received a loading dose of phenobarbitone (20 mg/kg). She was subsequently referred to the NICU. On admission she was breathing spontaneously, and she was irritable and hypertonic. She had a severe generalized tonic seizure upon admission.

The aEEG registration was immediately started showing ongoing seizure activity. Midazolam was given for clinical seizures (at asterisks) which correlated with aEEG discharges, with only a short-lasting effect. When the seizures recurred they were all subclinical and of short duration and the infant was still breathing spontaneously. Lidocaine was added to the medication but there was relentless ongoing seizure activity. Clonazepam was added to the medication overnight and because of apneas, she was eventually intubated and ventilated. Note the minimal lifting of the baseline during seizure activity.

Cranial ultrasound examination showed extensive areas of increased echogenicity in the basal ganglia as well as the white matter. As there was a discrepancy between the perinatal history and the clinical picture after the first 24 h, extensive additional metabolic investigations were performed, but these were all negative. Intensive care treatment was withdrawn. Permission for postmortem was obtained and extensive hypoxic–ischemic brain damage was found

65

5

Hypoxia–ischemia and aEEG

The neonatal EEG is depressed during and immediately after an acute hypoxic–ischemic insult[95–99]. The degree and duration of the EEG depression correlates with the severity of the brain injury[100,101]. During the recovery, the EEG subsequently contains information on the severity of the previous hypoxic–ischemic insult. In newborn infants, the electrocortical activity is a highly sensitive predictor of neurological outcome when recorded early after a hypoxic–ischemic insult[81,102–106]. Several studies have shown that outcome can be accurately predicted from an aEEG during the first hours of life[45,107–111].

In asphyxiated full-term infants, the aEEG can accurately predict outcome in 80% of the infants at 3 h and in 90% of the infants at 6 h postnatally[45,109,110]. The early aEEG background in asphyxiated infants correlates with the degree of HIE, with levels of neurone-specific enolase in the cerebrospinal fluid, and with cerebral glucose metabolism later in the neonatal period[46,112]. Preliminary data indicate that a combined approach including aEEG and clinical evaluation of HIE increases the predictive accuracy after asphyxia[113]. At present, the early aEEG is used for evaluation of babies before inclusion in postasphyctic intervention studies.

The electrocortical background activity is the most important factor for prediction of outcome. Presence of epileptic seizure activity does not seem to be as strong a predictor as the background activity. Seizures did not seem to affect outcome in asphyxiated infants with mild HIE or a normal EEG. However, seizures were correlated with worse outcome in infants with moderate to severe HIE or a low-voltage EEG[78,85]. Furthermore, the postnatal age when postasphyctic seizures develop could be correlated with outcome, although different results have been obtained[46,114]. Table 1 presents a summary of predictive features in aEEG from preliminary data[46].

Reactivity to caregiving is seen as a short transient rise in the aEEG background, when the aEEG is discontinuous and the infant is not too ill or heavily sedated (see Figure 2.9). Reactivity is not usually clearly discernible in infants with a CNV aEEG background, and this could be one reason why this feature was not associated with outcome (Table 1).

The electrocortical background normalizes and becomes CNV in most full-term infants within 1–2 weeks following a hypoxic–ischemic incident. After the first days, a standard EEG is better for evaluation of electrocortical abnormalities since the expected findings are subtler and sometimes not possible to detect with the aEEG, e.g. signs of dysmaturity or presence of positive rolandic sharp waves in preterm infants with periventricular leukomalacia (PVL)[81,97,115,116].

Critically ill and unstable neonates may experience several events during intensive care that may negatively affect brain function, e.g. periods with low or unstable oxygenation and blood pressure. With the aEEG it is possible to follow the impact on the brain from such events in both full-term and preterm infants, as shown in Figures 2.9c, 2.9d and 2.14 in Chapter 2 and 6.3 and 7.3 later in the Atlas. The ability of the aEEG to predict neurological outcome after hypoxic–ischemic events occurring later in the neonatal period has been little studied, although the scarce data indicate that the aEEG background and the recovery rate are correlated with outcome[103].

Table I Summary of the impact of different aEEG features for prediction of outcome in asphyxiated full-term infants. Modified from reference 46

	Hours		
Age	0–12	12–24	24–48
Background pattern	++	+	–
Epileptic seizures	–	+	–
Sleep–wake cycling	+	+	–
Reactivity to care	–	–	–

The EEG background in infants needing extra-corporeal membrane oxygenation (ECMO) seems to be predictive of neurological outcome, and subclinical seizure activity during ECMO treatment is not uncommon[60,117].

Burst suppression is usually a marker of severe brain damage in full-term infants and seems to constitute a disconnection in brain circuits between the cerebral cortex and deeper layers, e.g. the thalamus[118,119]. In asphyxiated fetal sheep, return of the EEG with a continuous low-voltage seizure pattern seems to be a marker of parasagittal injury[100,101]. Postmortem neuropathological investigations have shown a direct relationship between the number of damaged neurones and the EEG background activity in both full-term and premature infants[120,121]. Aso and colleagues found that EEG inactivity was correlated with widespread encephalomalacia engaging the cerebral cortex, corpus striatum, thalamus, midbrain and pons in postmortem studies of newborn infants[120]. Burst suppression was also related to multifocal severe brain damage but no damage to any specific brain structures were identified in these infants[120]. In asphyxiated piglets, the burst recovery (occurrence and duration) was predictive of outcome[122]. The finding that the burst rate after hypoxia–ischemia is related to later outcome is supported by a study in preterm infants with large germinal matrix–intraventricular hemorrhages (GMH–IVH). In these infants the burst rate during the first 48 h postnatally discriminated infants with poor outcome from those with fair outcome[123].

In asymmetrical cerebral lesions, e.g. middle cerebral artery infarction, concomitant asymmetry of the EEG background is common. It has been shown that the EEG background over the affected hemisphere is sensitive for prediction of later outcome, a normal background is predictive of normal outcome while an abnormal background increases the risk that the infant develops hemiplegia[124]. The aEEG has not been evaluated for this feature, although the asymmetry can been seen if the aEEG is recorded from more than one channel (see Figures 3.7 and 3.8). However, we do recommend that standard EEG and aEEG are combined in infants with clear asymmetrical cerebral lesions.

Neurological outcome is difficult to predict in extremely preterm infants during the first days of life. These infants anticipate a long neonatal intensive care period and several complications can occur that may compromise cerebral function, e.g. severe apnea and sepsis. Earlier studies suggested repeated EEG for prediction of outcome in these infants[125]. However, both the development of GMH–IVH and PVL is associated with a depressed EEG background and presence of epileptic seizure activity in very preterm infants. The degree of EEG depression is both related to the size of the hemorrhage and to the number of damaged brain structures (see Chapter 6)[39,61–63,121,123,126–129]. In preterm infants with a mean gestational age of 26 weeks, the aEEG during the first week of life had the same accuracy for prediction of outcome as cranial ultrasound[39]. In preterm infants with large GMH–IVH, crude outcome could be predicted by aEEG during the first 48 h of life[123]. Furthermore, sleep–wake cycling appearing in the aEEG during the first week of life was associated with better outcome in these infants.

Data reflecting the impact on the EEG from clear hypoxia–ischemia, such as PVL, are relatively scarce. Connell and colleagues found that the EEG depression often preceded ultrasound findings, both during development of GMH–IVH and PVL[32]. Epileptic seizure activity, often subclinical or with only subtle clinical manifestations, is relatively common during the development of GMH–IVH and PVL[39,61–63,126]. More recent data indicate that white-matter injury may be detected early by EEG monitoring that evaluates spectral-edge frequency[16].

- A CNV aEEG background, or a continuous but slightly periodic background pattern with normal amplitude, is predictive of good outcome in full-term infants;

- Abnormal aEEG patterns, including discontinuous patterns as burst-suppression and electrocerebral inactivity (i.e. flat), or extremely low-voltage patterns are predictive of poor outcome (death or severe handicap);

- Most asphyxiated infants with an early burst-suppression aEEG background have a poor neurological outcome. However, some infants with rapid recovery of the aEEG (during the first 24 h) survive without handicap[45,110];

- Almost all asphyxiated full-term infants with inactive or extremely low-voltage aEEG activity will die or develop severe handicap;

- Sedative and anticonvulsive medications can affect the aEEG background activity and contribute to a more uncertain evaluation of the aEEG pattern (see Chapter 2).

Mild HIE with good outcome

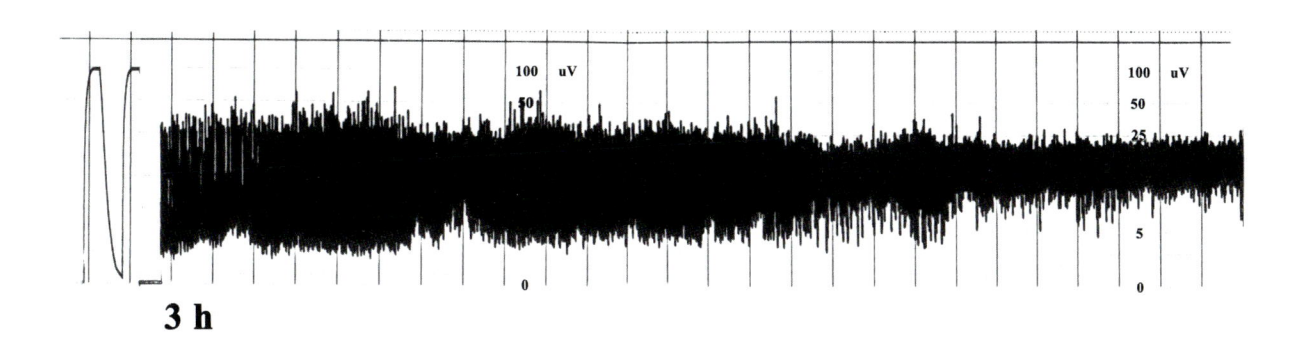

3 h

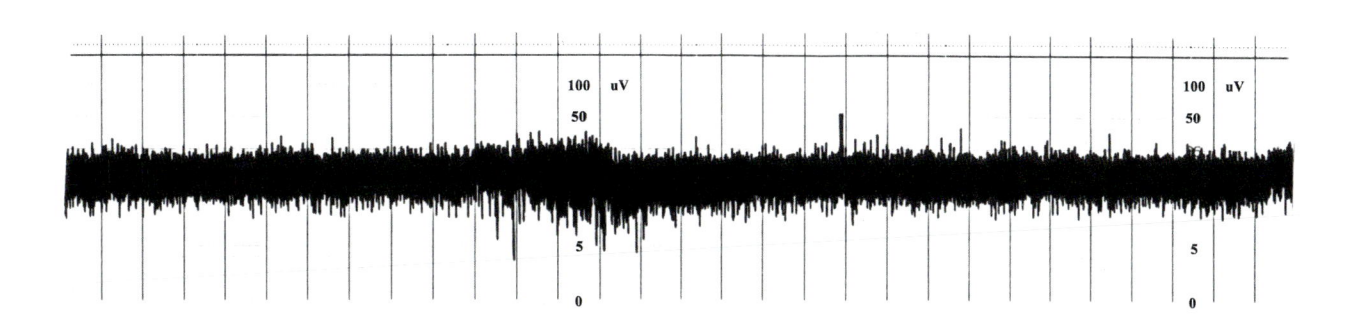

Figure 5.1 This male infant was born at 41 weeks' gestation following an uneventful pregnancy. During the delivery a persistent fetal bradycardia occurred which necessitated an emergency Cesarean section. The amniotic fluid was meconium-stained and he was intubated straight away. The Apgar scores were 3, 3 and 6 at 1, 5 and 10 min, respectively, and the umbilical arterial pH was 6.98. His birth weight was 3680 g. The recovery was rapid; he had only mild signs of encephalopathy and was extubated on day 2. Cranial ultrasound examination did not show any abnormalities and the infant had a normal neurodevelopmental outcome.

The aEEG tracing, recorded between 3 and 12 h of age, was initially discontinuous with a burst-suppression pattern. The cerebroelectrical background recovered rapidly over the next few hours from a DNV to a CNV pattern. At 9 h one cyclical period indicative of emerging sleep–wake cycling, was present (middle part of lower tracing).

This example shows an initially abnormal background at 3 h with rapid normalization to a CNV pattern within 6 h of age, predictive of a good outcome. The early emerging sleep–wake cycle is also predictive of a good outcome

Moderate HIE with signs of secondary energy failure

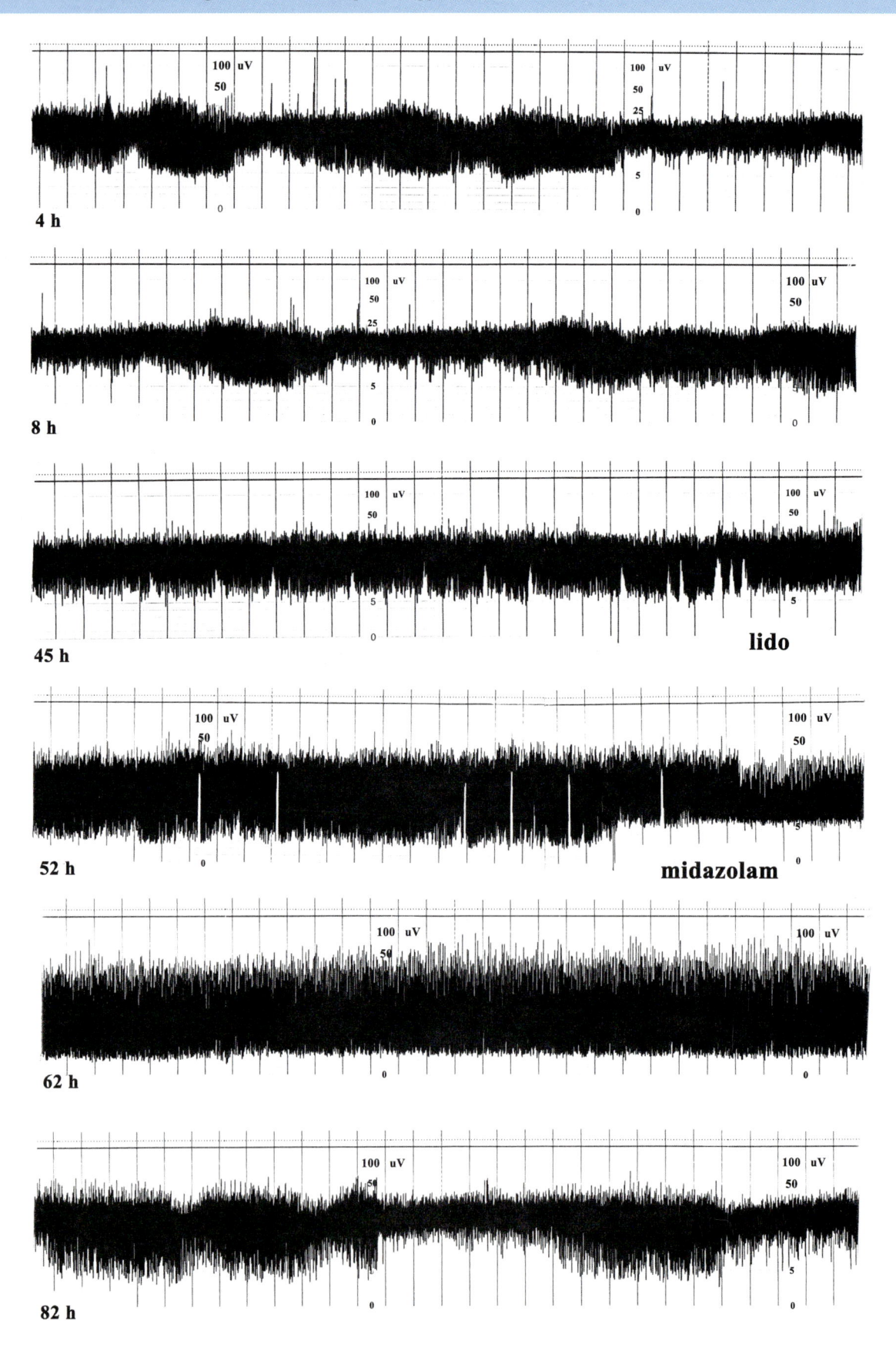

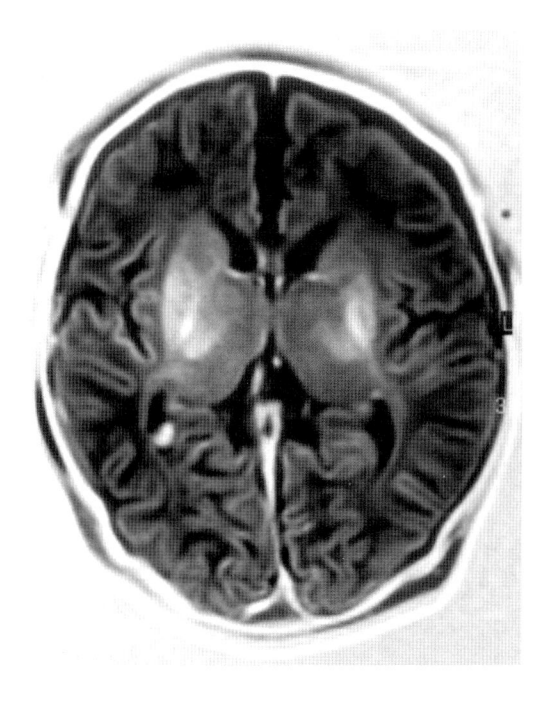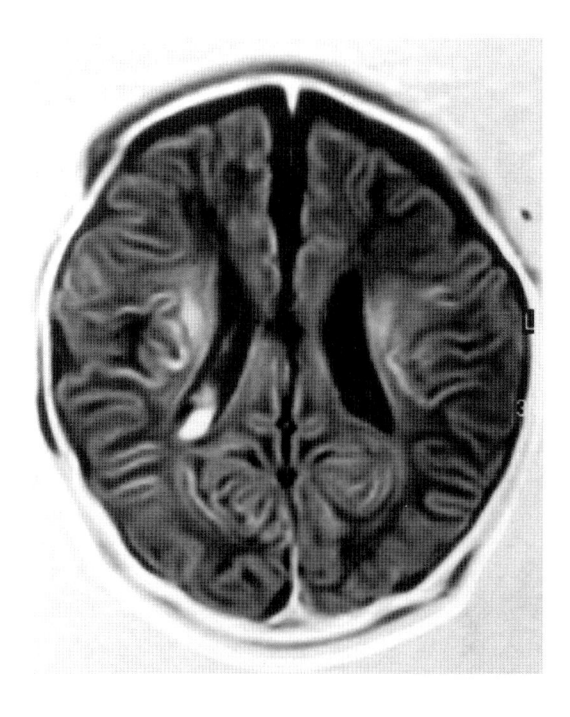

b

Figure 5.2 *opposite and above* This male infant was born at 41 weeks' gestation, following a normal vaginal delivery. His birth weight was 3400 g. He had an unexpectedly poor start, with Apgar scores 2, 4 and 4 at 1, 5 and 10 min, respectively. The umbilical arterial pH was 6.7 with a base excess of –25 mmol/l. He was intubated at 5 min of age and transferred to the NICU for further care. At 4 h his blood lactate was 11 mmol/l, but normalized within the first 24 h. He needed ventilatory support and required dopamine and dobutamine to sustain his blood pressure. When last seen at 18 months this boy showed a normal neurodevelopmental outcome with a developmental quotient of 111.

(a) The aEEG was started at 4 h of age. Initially, a CNV background pattern was seen as well as sleep–wake cycling. However, when the infant was 45 h old clinical seizures developed with corresponding recurrent epileptic seizure activity in the aEEG. Lidocaine (lido) was given with a good effect to start with, but electrographic seizures recurred at 53 h of age. The aEEG background became more discontinuous and the sleep–wake cycling was lost. Midazolam was added to the medication and no further epileptic seizures were seen in the aEEG. The background activity took some time to recover, with sleep–wake cycling restarting at 82 h of age. Reproduced from reference 53 with permission.

(b) MRI with inversion recovery sequence was performed at the end of the first week and shows a mild increase in signal intensity in the thalami and basal ganglia, and a small GMH–IVH on the right side. A normal signal was obtained from the posterior limb of the internal capsule, which is associated with good outcome[130].

This is an example of initial recovery with suspected secondary energy failure presenting with seizures and deterioration of electrocortical background activity. It also shows the importance of prolonged registration, even when the initial aEEG is reassuring

Moderate HIE with fair outcome

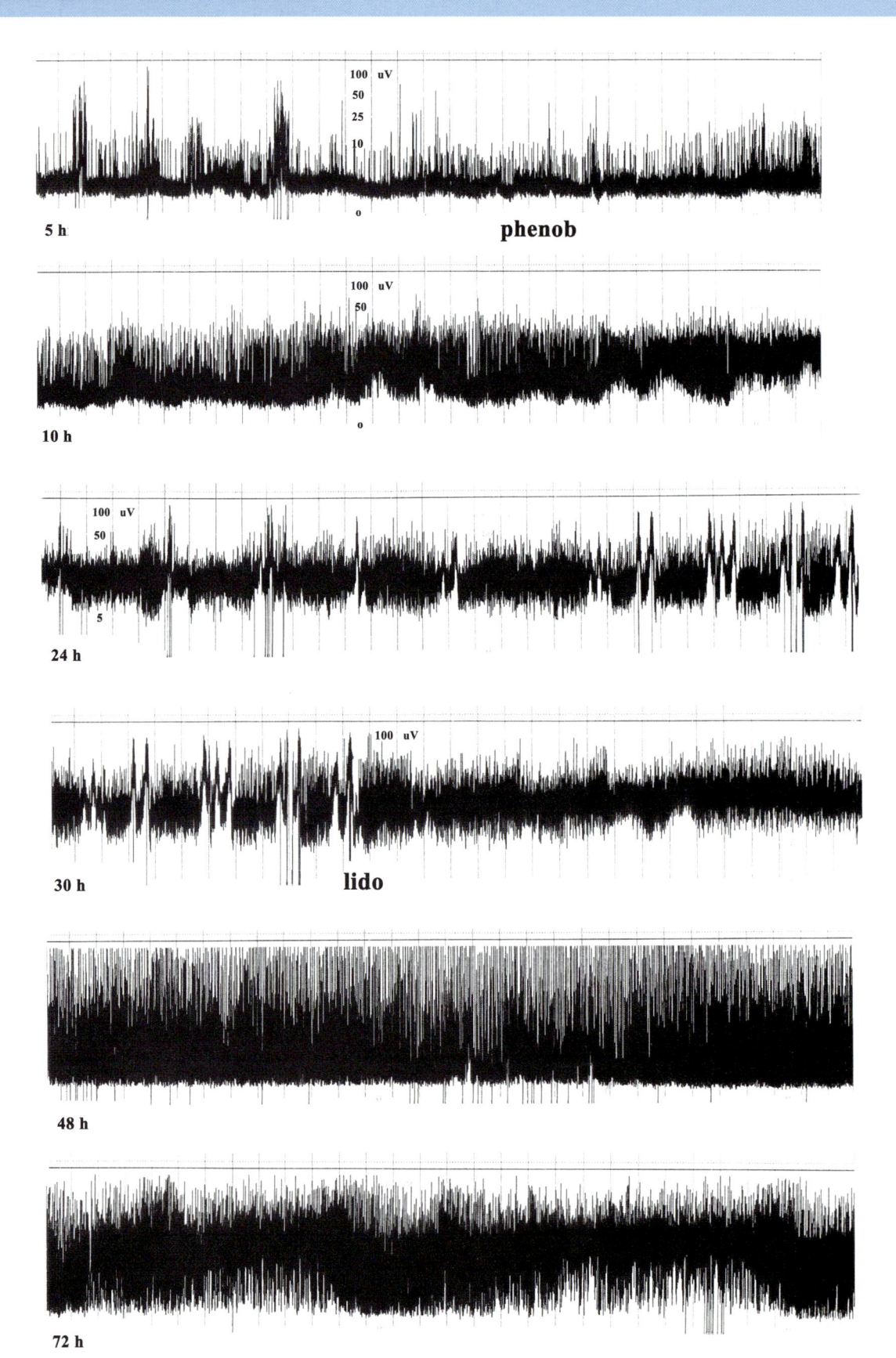

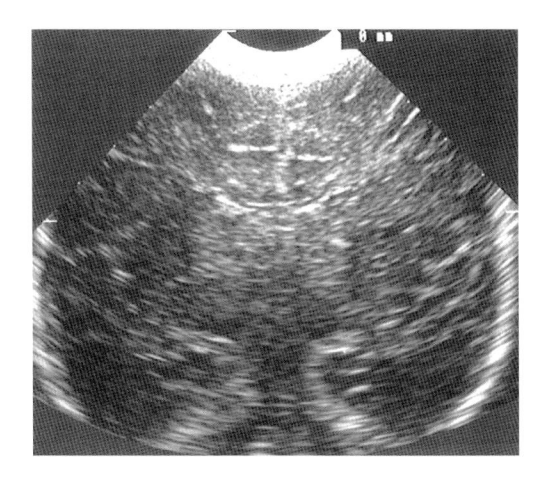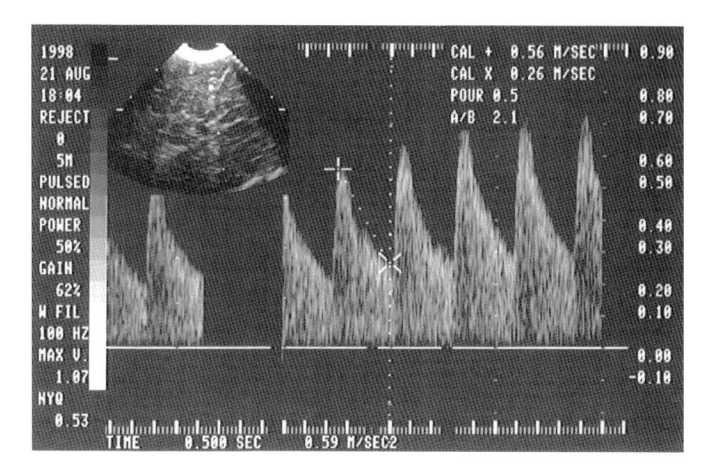

b

Figure 5.3 *opposite and above* The mother of this male infant had preterm rupture of the membranes and the delivery was induced. Fetal bradycardia and vaginal hemorrhage occurred after administration of oxytocine and led to an emergency Cesarean section at 41 weeks' gestation. Apgar scores were 1, 2 and 2 at 1, 5 and 10 min, respectively, and the birth weight was 2950 g. He was intubated and resuscitated, including cardiac massage and several doses of endotracheal adrenaline. A good heart rate was first noted at 14 min. The first capillary pH at 30 min was 6.93 with a base excess of –20 mmol/l. Clinical seizures were first seen at 2.5 h of age and phenobarbitone (phenob; 15 mg/kg) was given. He was then referred to the regional NICU. On admission, the arterial lactate level was 13.4 mmol/l but decreased to 2.6 mmol/l at 12 h of age. He required mild ventilatory support for a few days, and dopamine to support the blood pressure. Ultrasound and MRI showed abnormalities in the thalami. The posterior limb of the internal capsule on MRI, however, showed a normal signal. At 24 months of age he had a mild abnormality in tone, but was already able to take a few steps on his own, and had a developmental quotient of 95.

(a) The aEEG was started at 5 h of age and showed a very depressed burst-suppression pattern, almost flat. At 8 h of age, another 5 mg/kg of phenobarbitone was given in order to reach a usual loading of 20 mg/kg. No depressive effect was seen from the extra phenobarbitone on the aEEG, which slowly and gradually improved – initially in burst density and later in amplitude. At 24 h of age the background activity was continuous but at this stage, a seizure pattern developed. The epileptic seizure activity continued for several hours and stopped following administration of lidocaine (lido). During the following hours the background activity became discontinuous and changed to a dense burst-suppression pattern at 48 h of age. The aEEG background gradually improved again, but was still abnormal at 72 h, although it showed some variability suggestive of emerging sleep–wake cycling.

(b) Cranial ultrasound was performed on day 3; the coronal view shows mild increase in echogenicity in the thalami. A Doppler signal obtained from the middle cerebral artery showed increased diastolic flow, indicating poor outcome[131].

This infant is a good example of the insight into brain function that is obtained when continuous aEEG recording is performed from shortly after birth for a prolonged period of time. The aEEG depression during the second day of life could be due either to brain injury or to the administered antiepileptic medication, or both

Moderate HIE with poor outcome

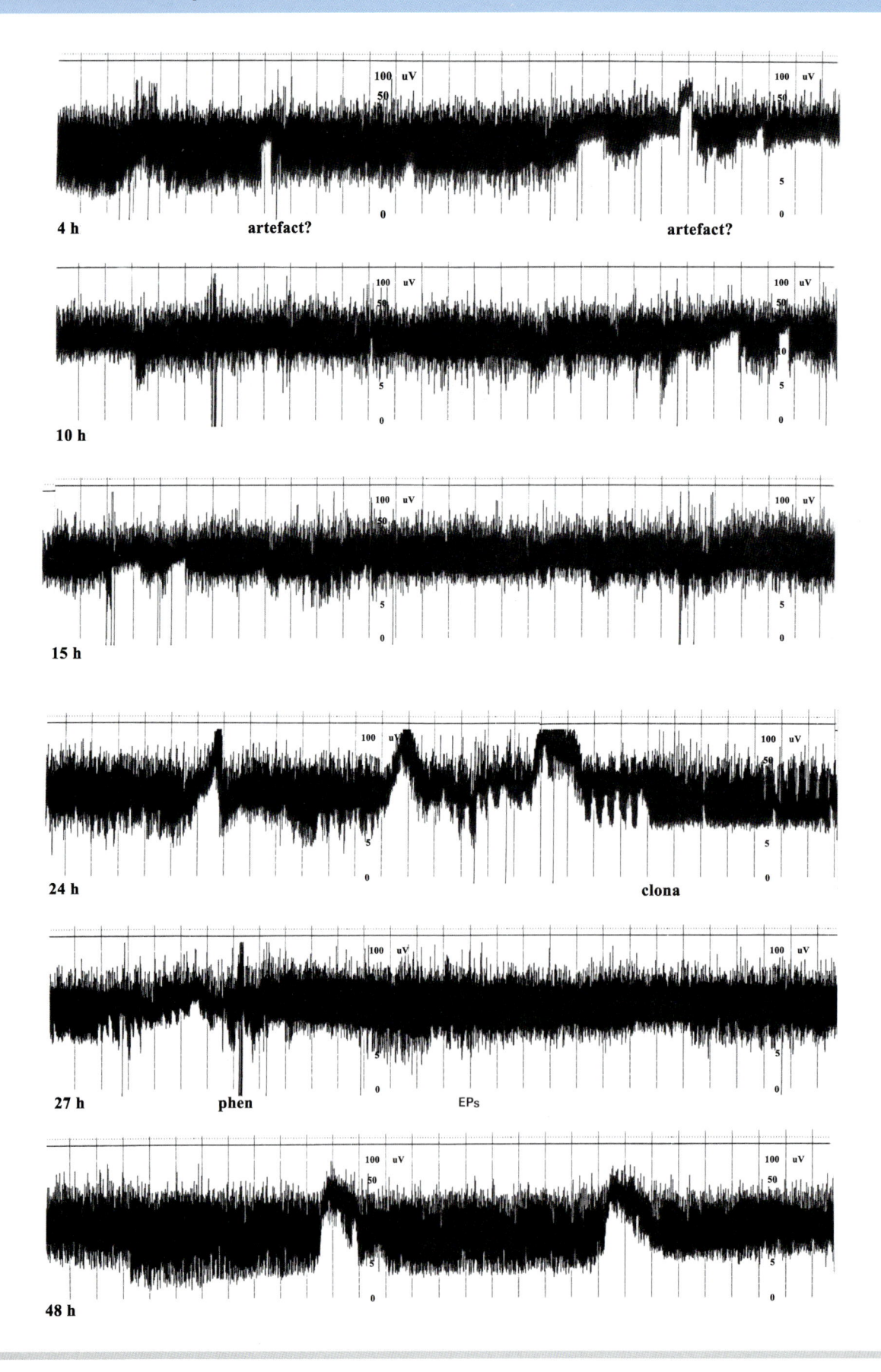

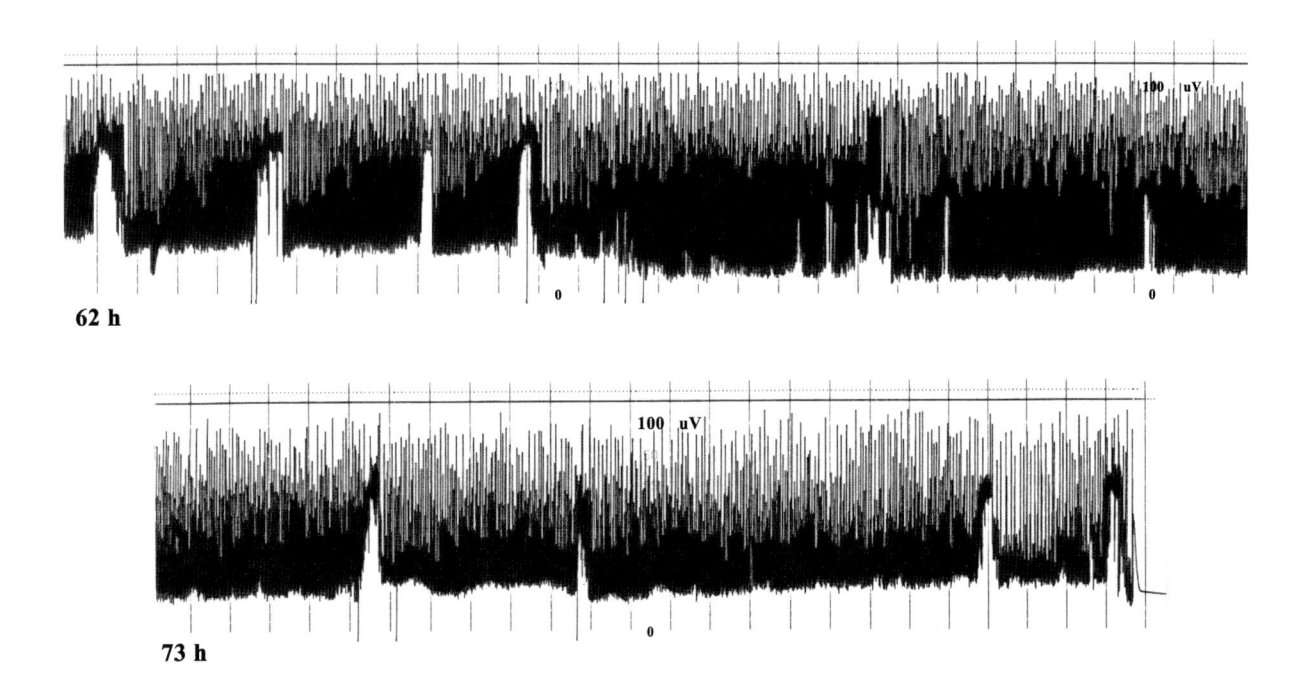

Figure 5.4 *opposite and above* This asphyxiated male infant was delivered at 41 weeks' gestation. The amniotic fluid was heavily meconium-stained, the umbilical pH was 6.95 and Apgar scores were 4, 6 and 8 at 1, 5 and 10 min, respectively. He was immediately intubated and large amounts of meconium were suctioned from below the vocal cords. After 10 min he needed reintubation as the tube became blocked with thick meconium. The infant was transferred to the NICU; the arterial lactate level was 12.5 mmol/l on arrival. He required high-ventilation pressures and 100% oxygen, and immediately following admission he was changed to high-frequency oscillation ventilation. He also received surfactant and nitrous oxide, but neither had a positive effect. He was paralyzed and required 100% oxygen until he died. He also required large doses of inotropic support, including dopamine, dobutamine and corticosteroids. He was given antibiotics, but only the skin culture grew group B streptococci; all other cultures were negative.

When he was 4 days old cranial ultrasound showed extensive areas of increased echogenicity in the periventricular and subcortical white matter. SEPs could not be elicited. Intensive care treatment was withdrawn, because of severe pulmonary and neurological problems. Permission for postmortem examination was obtained and histology of the brain showed extensive areas of hypoxic–ischemic damage.

The aEEG was started immediately following admission as the infant had suffered perinatal asphyxia and also because he was paralyzed for optimal ventilation. A DNV background pattern was seen and a first suspected single seizure was noted shortly after starting the registration (marked 'artefact?'). Phenobarbitone was given, but a few more suspected seizures with the same appearance were seen on the tracings beginning at 10 and 15 h. In spite of his illness and the phenobarbitone, the background activity recovered and became continuous with normal voltage.

During the second day (trace beginning at 24 h) two types of seizure patterns were seen in the aEEG: three seizures of 10–15-min duration with transient rises in both minimum and maximum amplitudes, and several shorter seizures of 2–3-min duration and changes only in the minimum amplitudes. A loading dose of clonazepam (clona) at 28 h seemed to abolish seizure activity for 45 min, although during the last 30 min of the tracing suspected short seizure activity with regularly recurring decreases in the maximum amplitudes appeared. Phenytoin (phen) was added when the infant was 28 h (trace beginning at 27 h), and appeared to stop the seizure activity until 48 h of age. At that time new seizure activity appeared; the trace beginning at 48 h shows two seizures each with a 15-min duration. The background activity was moderately depressed and became more discontinuous. At 62 h of age, recurrent seizures of 2–5-min duration appeared on a burst-suppression background and continued until the end of the recording.

This example shows the importance of using aEEG in infants who are paralyzed when ventilated. It also shows the need for longer registrations, as the seizures became more frequent after the first day of life and the background started to deteriorate after the second day of life

Moderate HIE and survival with poor outcome

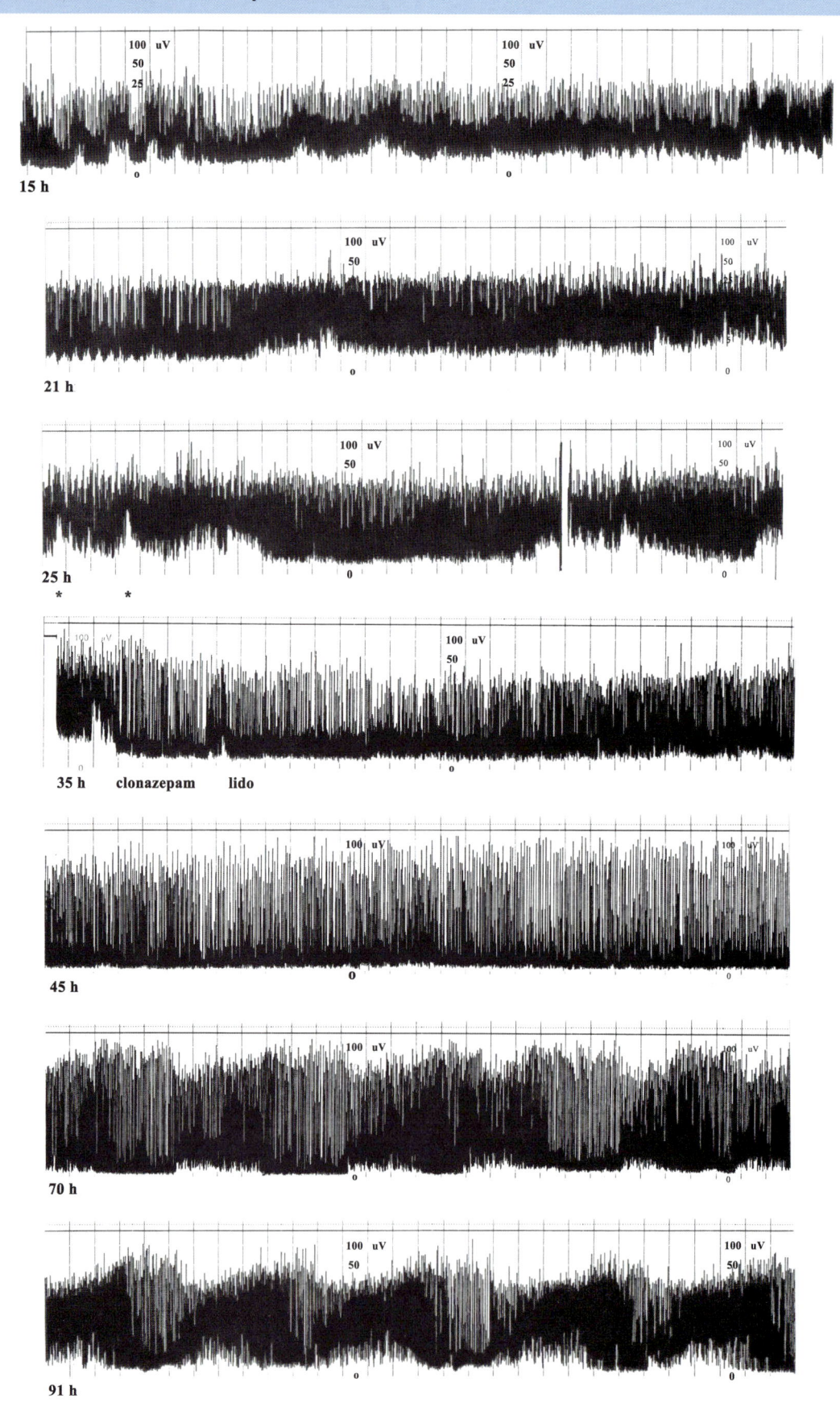

15 h

21 h

25 h
*   *

35 h   clonazepam   lido

45 h

70 h

a

91 h

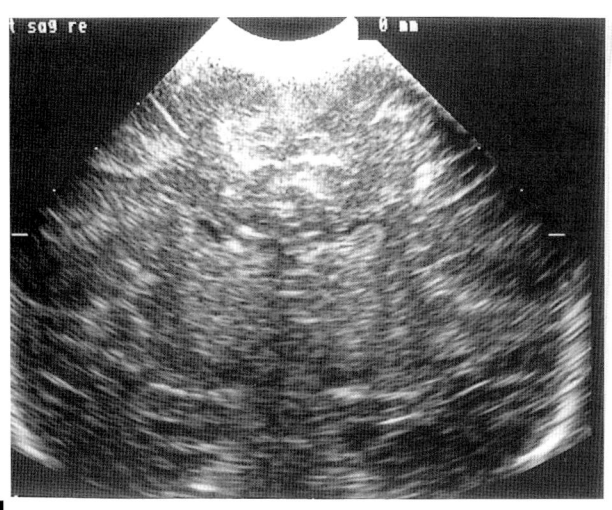
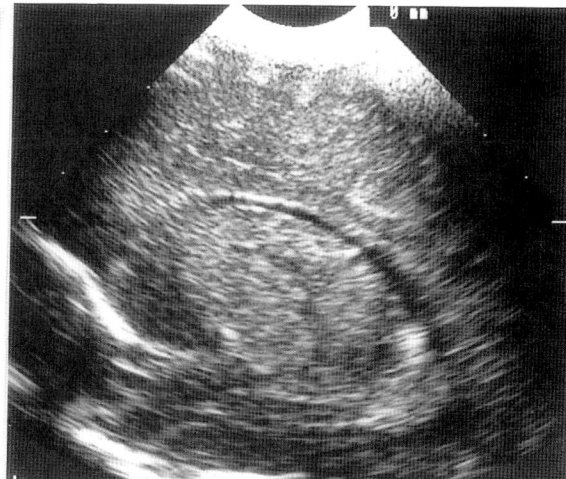

b

Figure 5.5 *opposite and above* This female infant was born at 40 weeks' gestation following an emergency Cesarean section due to placental abruption. The umbilical arterial pH was 6.68. She had a poor start with Apgar scores 1, 3 and 4 at 1, 5 and 10 min, respectively. She was immediately intubated and ventilated and a good heart rate was first present at 7 min. After the initial resuscitation she was stable and required mechanical ventilation only for the first 12 h. Ultrasound and MRI showed extensive abnormalities in the basal ganglia, with a reversed signal of the posterior limb of the internal capsule on MRI. A focal area of cystic subcortical leukomalacia also developed in the left parietal region. At 3 years her outcome was severely abnormal with quadriplegia, microcephaly, mental retardation and cerebral visual impairment.

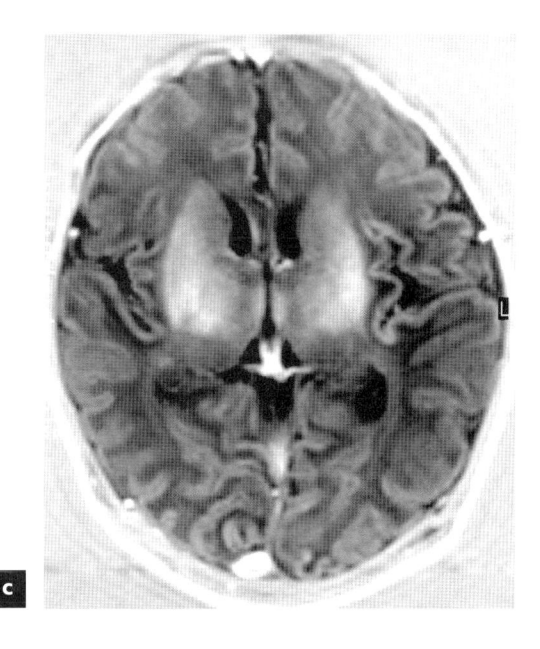

c

(a) The aEEG was started at 15 h of age and shows a discontinuous burst-suppression-like background pattern with relatively low amplitude. Four suspected seizures are seen at the beginning of the recording as transient rises in the minimum amplitude of 5–10-min duration. Again, (at the end of the tracing beginning at 15 h) at around 18 h suspected recurrent seizure activity with short duration is appearing as a 'saw-tooth' pattern in the minimum amplitude. The suspected seizure pattern continued during most of the next tracing (beginning at 21 h) and until 25 h when she also had two clinical seizures (at asterisks). A slight recovery of the background activity can be seen during the first 30 h, with increased burst density and increased burst amplitude, although no major change occurred in the burst-suppression background pattern. She did not receive any antiepileptic treatment until later when clonazepam and lidocaine (lido) were administered (tracing starting at 35 h). The background pattern again became more depressed after the antiepileptic treatment. No subsequent seizure activity was noted. Some variability in the background activity first occurred at 70 h of age, but at 91 h this had still not developed to a normal sleep–wake cycling pattern.

The slow recovery of the aEEG background in this infant was predictive of poor neurological outcome. Since she did not receive antiepileptic medications until later, it is obvious that the lack of background recovery was due to the brain injury.

(b) Cranial ultrasound was performed at the end of the first week and showed areas of increased echogenicity in the thalamus and the basal ganglia in the coronal and parasagittal views. (c) The MRI, using inversion recovery sequence, showed lack of normal myelination in the posterior limb of the internal capsule and areas of increased signal intensity in the basal ganglia and thalami when this infant was 1 week old

Discrepancy between clinical behavior and aEEG

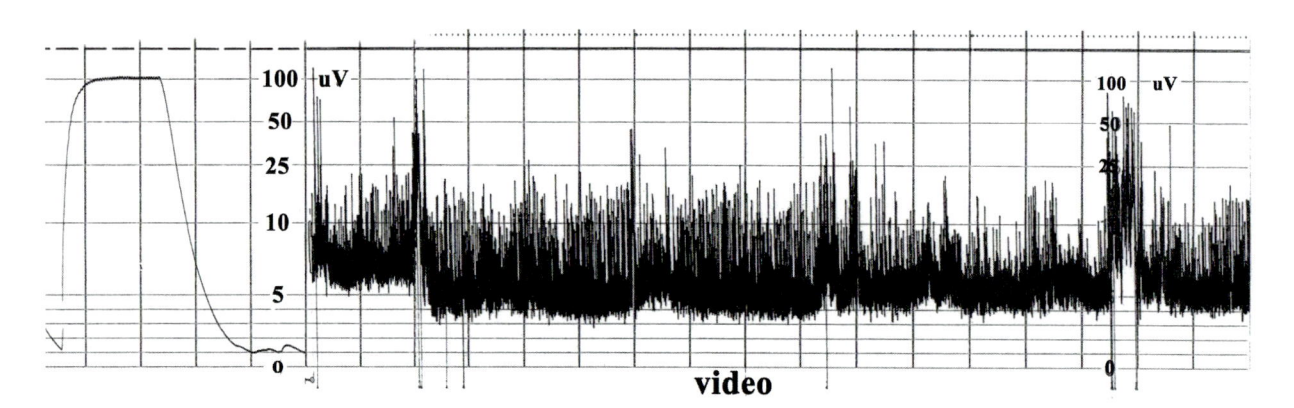

10 h

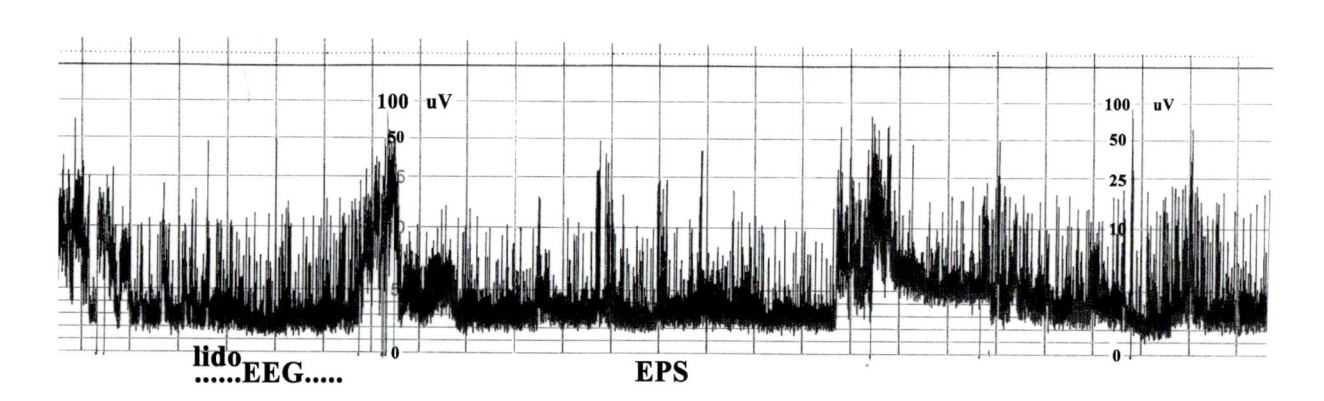

14 h

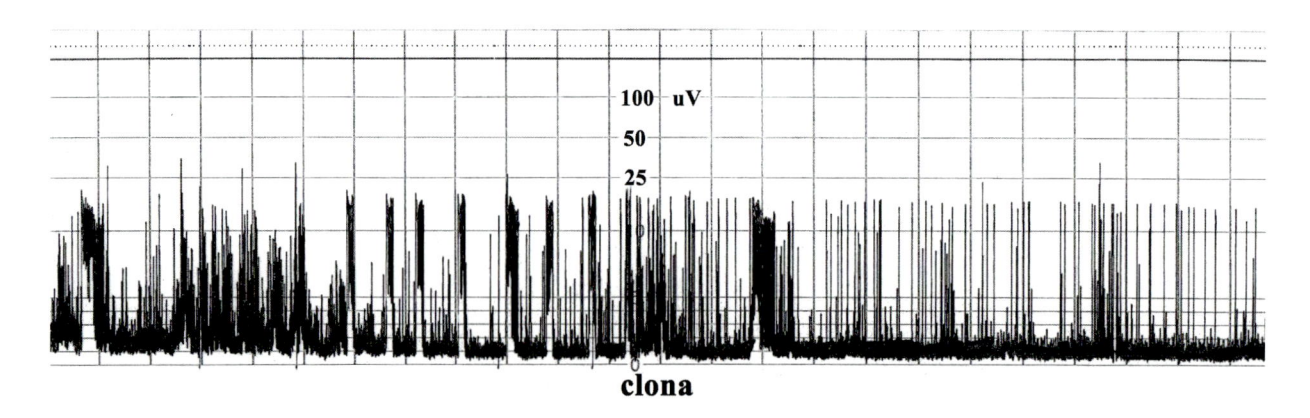

21 h

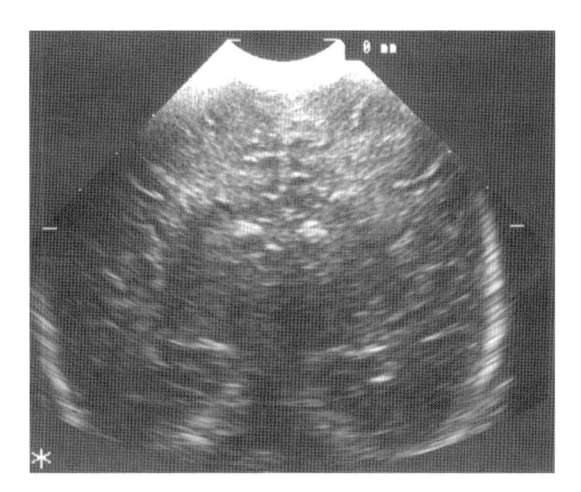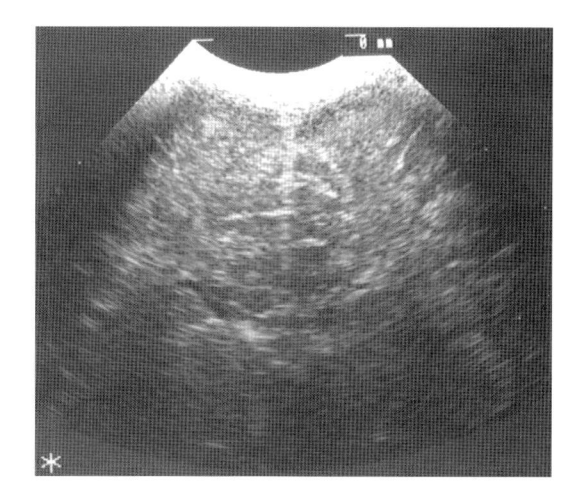

Figure 5.6 *opposite and above* Clinical behavior is not always reliable in the evaluation after birth asphyxia. This male twin was born at 38 weeks' gestation, after a pregnancy complicated by twin–twin transfusion syndrome (TTTS). The delivery was initially induced, but since the cardiotocograph of this twin was lost all of a sudden an emergency Cesarean section was performed. The infant was depressed at birth and briefly hand bagged, following which regular spontaneous ventilation was established. His Apgar scores were 2, 6 and 8 at 1, 5 and 10 min, respectively. The umbilical arterial pH was 6.78 and a first arterial lactate level was 23 mmol/l and remained elevated over the following 12 h. His birth weight was 2300 g; the other twin weighed 3300 g. At 24 h he developed severe apneas and mechanical ventilation was started. At 36 h of age he suddenly developed a persistent bradycardia and died in spite of resuscitation. Cranial ultrasound (coronal views using a 7.5- (left) and a 10-MHz (right) transducer) showed diffuse increased echogenicity of the periventricular and deep white matter suggestive of fetal distress of longer duration.

The aEEG was started immediately following admission. The aEEG showed a discontinuous burst-suppression pattern of relatively low amplitude with the minimum amplitude at 3–4 μV. The zero baseline had been calibrated to the 1-μV level, but this has no impact on the basic aEEG pattern and very little effect on the amplitude. The child was sucking a dummy at this time and was responsive to handling (and was video recorded).

In the beginning of the second trace a suspected seizure pattern is present. This was confirmed somewhat later by a standard EEG that showed short runs of electrical discharges of 10–20-s duration. The seizure pattern in the aEEG meanwhile, when the EEG was recorded, can be suspected but is difficult to be certain about. Lidocaine (lido) was given and the electrographic seizures disappeared. The two transient increases in the aEEG amplitude, each of 10–20-min duration, were due to movement artefacts. EPs were performed which were delayed and low in amplitude (suggestive of poor outcome when still delayed after the first 3–4 days of life)[132].

Later (bottom tracing), from about 24 h, again a seizure pattern recurred on a severely depressed burst-suppression background. After clonazepam (clona) one suspected seizure with 2–3-min duration can be seen; otherwise the aEEG background shows a severely depressed burst-suppression pattern.

The discrepancy between the initial clinical behavior and the aEEG background and outcome is unusual. The abnormal aEEG predicted the poor outcome in spite of the clinical behavior

Severe HIE with poor outcome

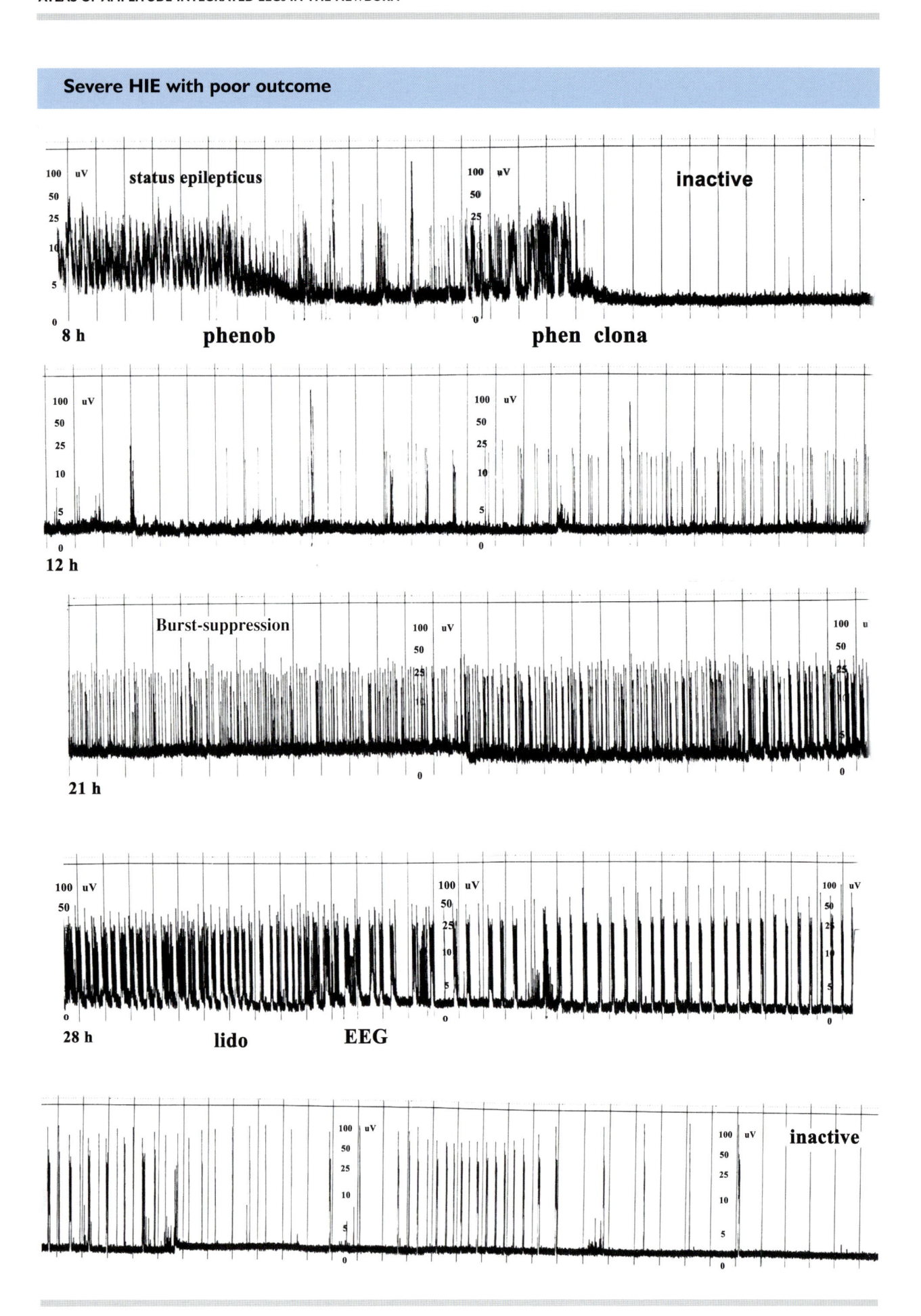

Figure 5.7 *opposite*   This female infant was born at term following a planned home delivery. Her birth weight was 3870 g. The amniotic fluid was heavily meconium-stained and she made only small efforts to breathe. She was transported to the local hospital where she was briefly ventilated using bag and mask. Her first capillary blood sample at 1 h of age showed a pH of 7.11 and a base excess of –11 mmol/l. Over the next hours, her oxygen requirements increased and she was intubated and ventilated. A chest X-ray showed signs of severe meconium aspiration. At that stage she was transferred to the regional NICU. On arrival, she was making extensive rowing movements and was lip-smacking. Cranial ultrasound showed areas of increased echogenicity in the thalami. An MRI, performed on day 4, confirmed these findings and proton spectroscopy showed large lactate peaks in these areas.

The aEEG was started following admission at 8 h (upper trace), and initially showed a 'saw-tooth' pattern corresponding with status epilepticus. The epileptic seizure activity stopped following administration of phenobarbitone (phenob; 20 mg/kg intravenously), and the background became profoundly depressed and mainly inactive. One hour later, seizures recurred. Phenytoin (phen; 15 mg/kg intravenously) and clonazepam (clona; 0.1 mg/kg intravenously) were given and resulted in an entirely flat trace for several hours.

A burst-suppression pattern gradually appeared (second and third tracings) with increasing burst density, but still severely abnormal.

On the fourth tracing, at 28 h of age the seizure pattern again evolved into a subclinical status epilepticus with short seizures on a severely depressed background. Lidocaine (lido) was given but had little effect on the seizure pattern, although 1 h later the interictal interval increased from 2 min to 5 min. A standard EEG confirmed the epileptic seizure activity. After some hours the aEEG background eventually became entirely flat. At that stage it was decided to discontinue intensive care treatment.

The initial aEEG in this asphyxiated infant with meconium aspiration and abnormal neurology, was severely abnormal with early seizure activity and a severely depressed background. The early abnormal aEEG is predictive of poor outcome and is confirmed by the lack of normalization of the electrocortical background during the first days of life, and the abnormal ultrasound and MRI investigations

Severe birth asphyxia in a moderately preterm infant

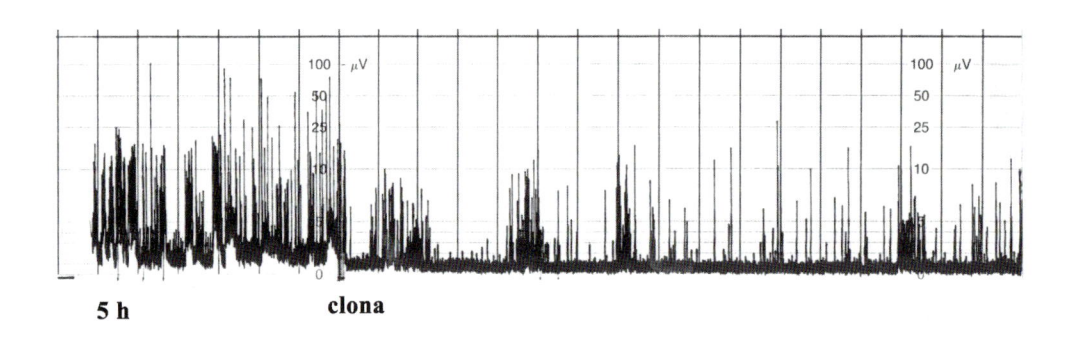

5 h   clona

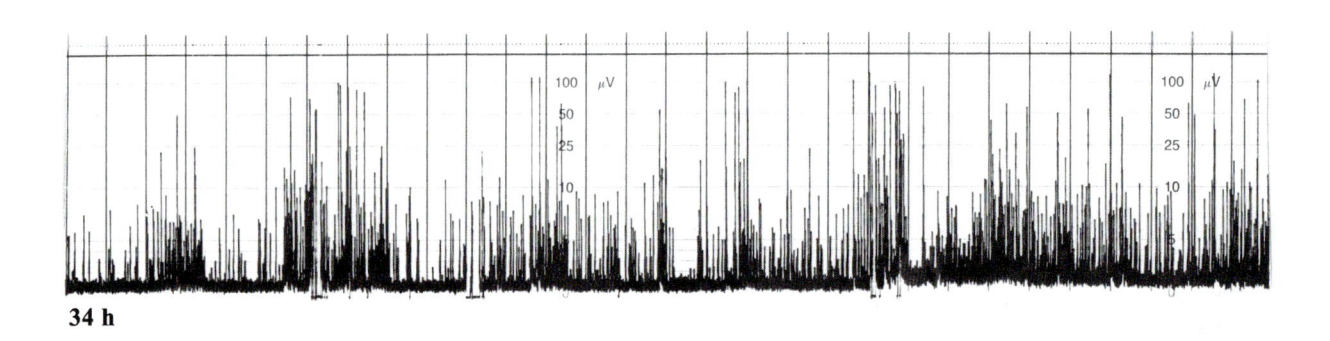

34 h

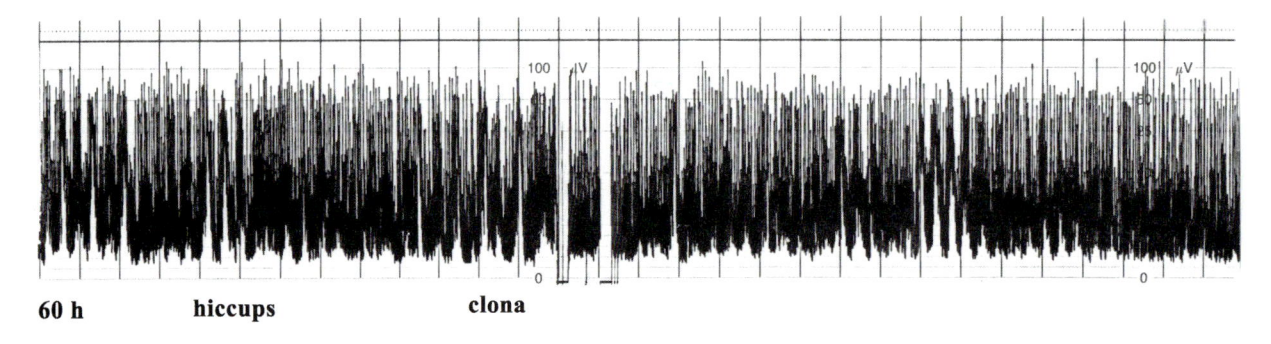

60 h   hiccups   clona

a

Figure 5.8   This female infant was born as the first of twins at 33 weeks' gestation, following preterm rupture of the membrane and signs of maternal infection. She was severely asphyxiated at birth with Apgar scores of 0, 0 and 2 at 1, 5 and 10 min, respectively. She was intubated and ventilated. The first capillary pH at 20 min of age was 6.78 with a base excess of –20 mmol/l. On admission at the regional NICU, she required little ventilation but had a large subcutaneous hematoma and showed little spontaneous movement. Her hemoglobin was only 6.3 mmol/l and she required dopamine to maintain her blood pressure.

(a) The aEEG was started at 5 h of age. A short seizure pattern on a depressed background was already present at the beginning of the recording. Clonazepam (clona) was administered and was effective in stopping the seizure activity. The electrocortical background activity became flat and remained mainly inactive for the following 24 h. Some low-amplitude bursts (exceeding 5 μV) of activity are seen with 5–20-min intervals. At 34 h (middle trace) the background activity had somewhat recovered but was still mainly inactive with some periodic burst activity. At 60 h (bottom trace), a seizure pattern reappeared with repetitive seizures of 2–3-min duration. The infant did not have any clinical seizures but had a period with hiccups that could represent seizures. Clonazepam was administered once again but had little effect on the seizures

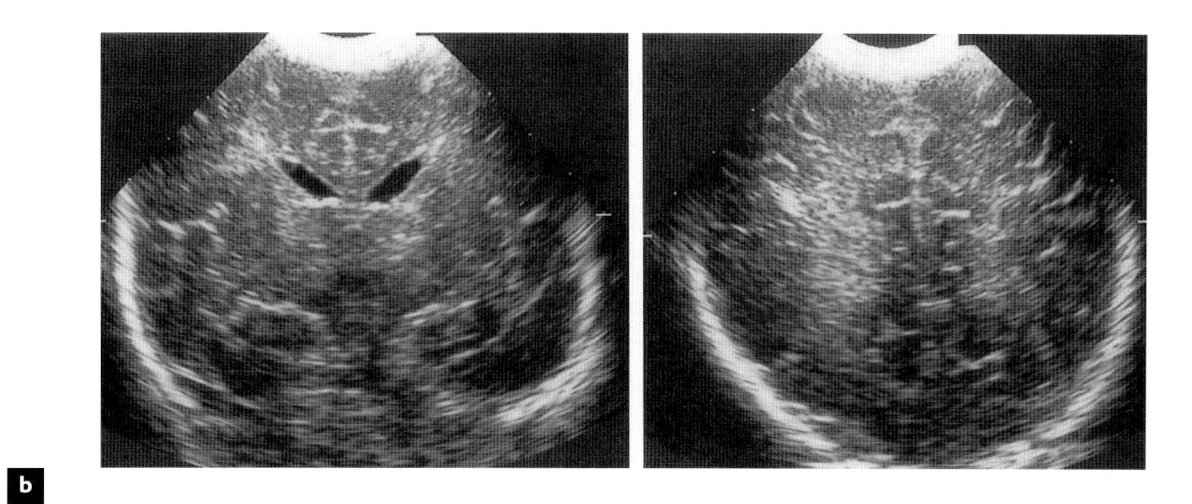

Figure 5.8 continued (b) A cranial ultrasound scan showed periventricular echogenicity, as well as symmetric mild echogenicity in the thalami, which can be seen in infants who suffer acute near total asphyxia. Her clinical condition did not improve and she developed clinical and subclinical seizures. Repeat cranial ultrasound investigations showed increased echogenicity in the thalami and in the periventricular white matter, and intensive care treatment was withdrawn.

The accuracy of the aEEG to predict outcome in asphyxiated preterm infants has not been evaluated. The severely abnormal and depressed background activity in this infant indicates poor outcome

Severe birth asphyxia in a preterm infant

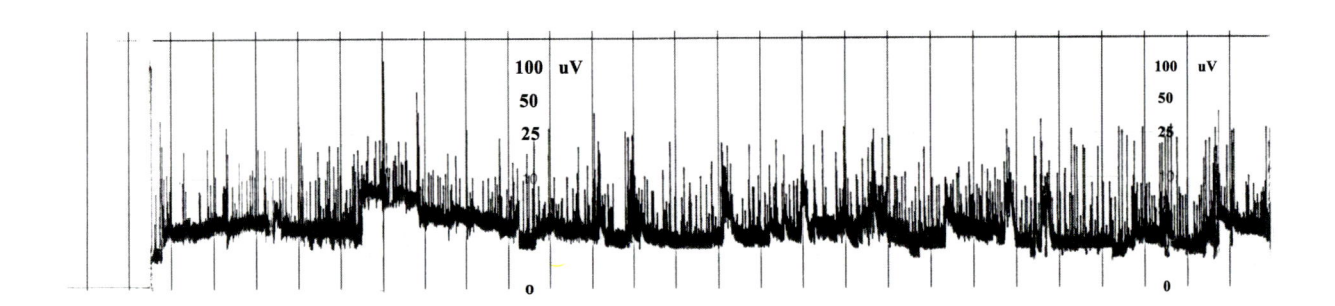

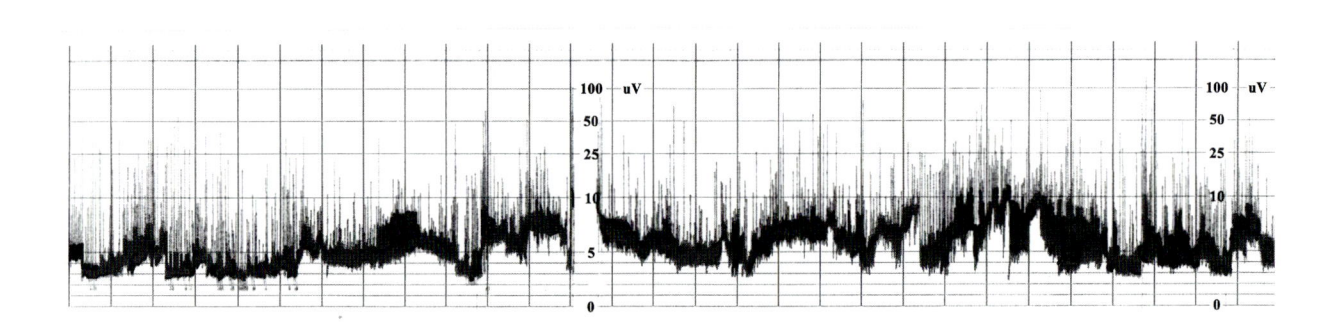

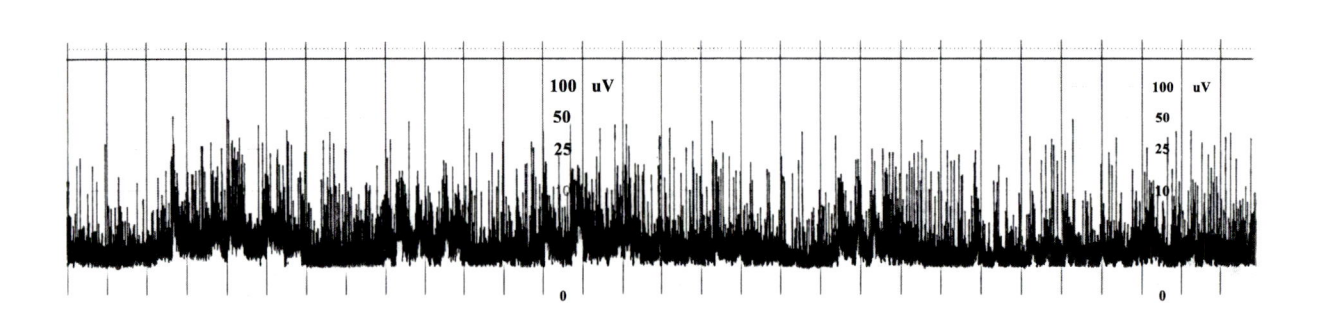

Figure 5.9 *opposite*   The mother of this male infant had mild hypertension at 30 weeks' gestation and developed abdominal pain. On arrival at the hospital the fetal heart rate was 30 beats/min. An emergency Cesarean section was performed and the diagnosis of placental abruption was confirmed. The baby weighed 1660 g. His Apgar scores were 0 at 1, 2 at 5 and 4 at 10 min. He was intubated and resuscitated with endotracheal adrenaline and cardiac massage. His heart rate only recovered after 30 min. The umbilical pH was 6.7, with a base excess of –28 mmol/l and a first arterial lactate level of 22.8 mmol/l. He was transferred to the tertiary-level NICU. He developed severe respiratory and circulatory problems and received surfactant, high-frequency oscillation ventilation and inotropic support with high doses of dopamine, dobutamine and hydrocortisone.

A cranial ultrasound scan showed a mild increase in periventricular echogenicity, but was otherwise unremarkable. Visual and somatosensory evoked potentials could not be obtained. In spite of the intensive care treatment the infant died on the second day due to cardiovascular problems.

The aEEG was started following admission at 3 h of age. The aEEG background was initially mainly flat but changed into a low-amplitude burst-suppression pattern. The aEEG minimum amplitude (baseline) is somewhat variable between 3 and 5 µV. This is sometimes seen in infants with a very poor electrocortical background, and it is possible that this reflects recording of extracerebral activity. Suspected recurrent seizure activity is present in both traces, with transient short elevations of both minimum and maximum amplitudes at 5–30-min intervals.

As in the previous example the severely abnormal and depressed background activity in this preterm infant indicates poor outcome

Localized PVL in a preterm infant

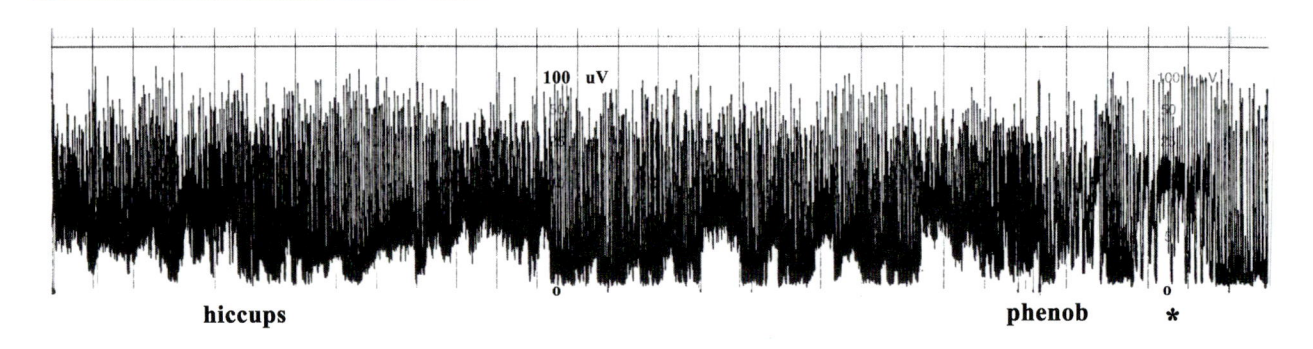

hiccups   phenob   *

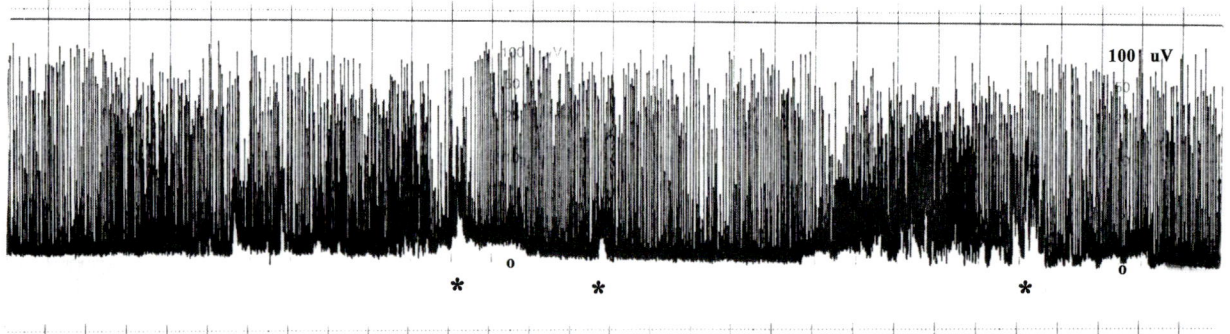

*   *   *

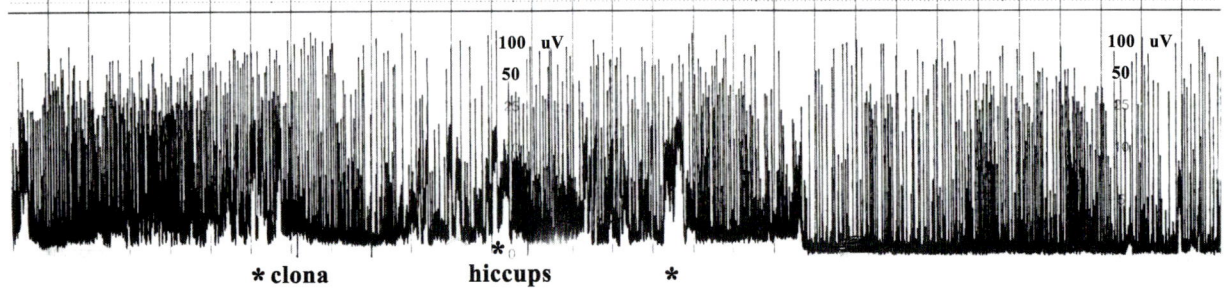

* clona   hiccups   *

a

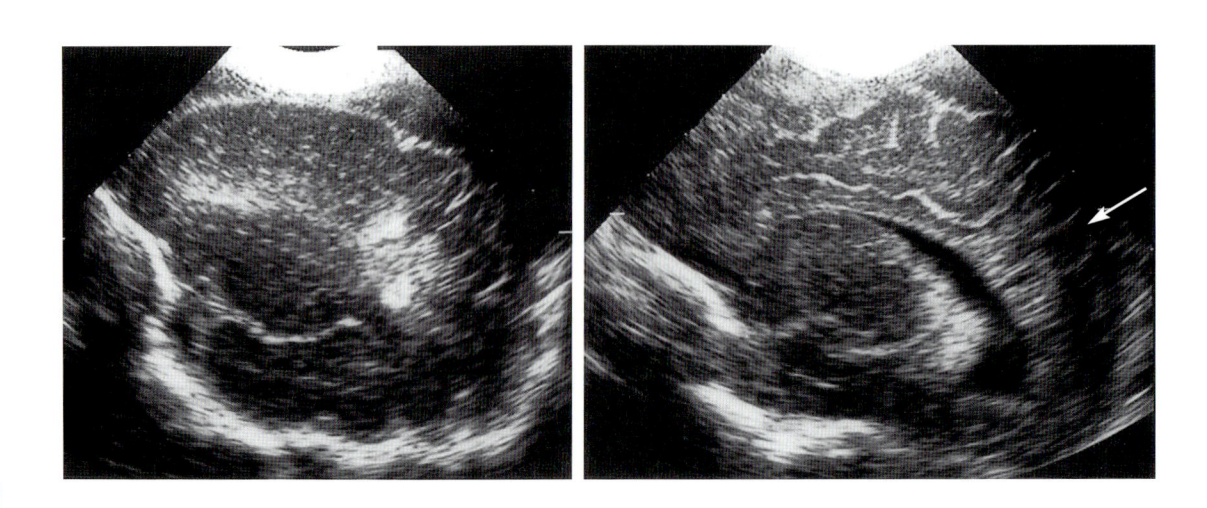

b

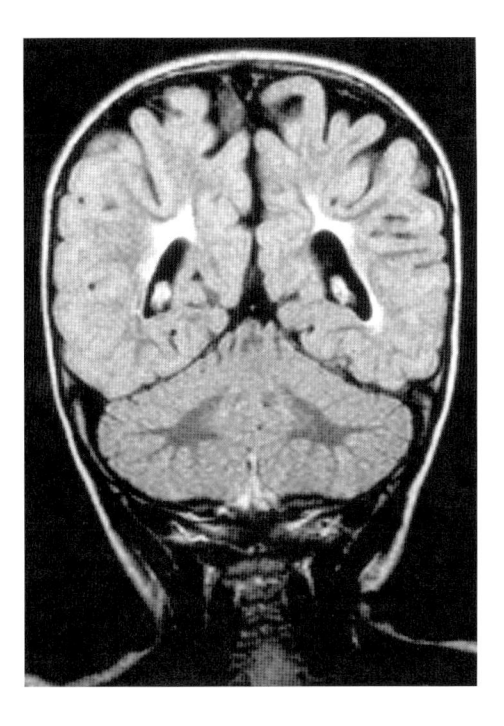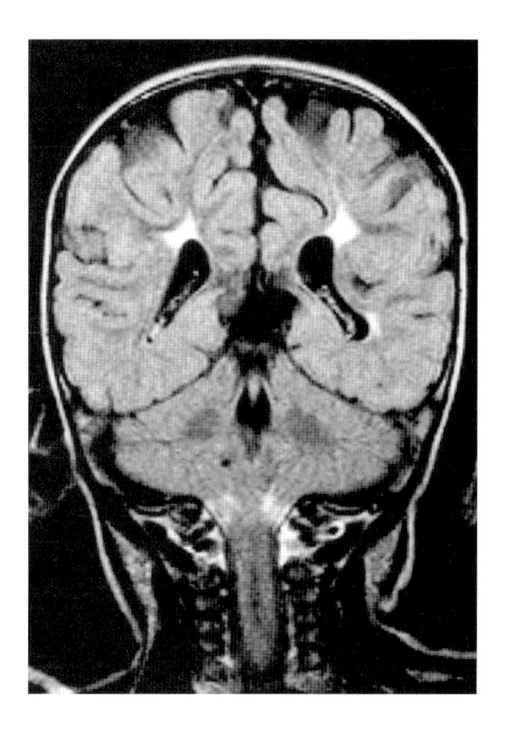

c

Figure 5.10 *opposite and above*   This male infant was the second of twins born at 29 weeks' gestation, by vaginal breech delivery and following 20 h of ruptured membranes. His Apgar scores were 6 at 1 min and 8 at 5 min. His birth weight was 1820 g. Shortly after delivery he developed respiratory distress and was intubated and ventilated. He was then transferred to the regional NICU. He required inotropic support to maintain the blood pressure, and received indomethacin for a persistent ductus arteriosus. The blood culture was negative, but all skin swabs were positive for *Staphylococcus aureus* for which he received treatment.

The initial cranial ultrasound scan showed mild periventricular echogenicity. On day 5, a small left-sided GMH–IVH was seen for the first time and associated with an area of increased echogenicity in the periventricular white matter. At 3 weeks of age he had developed a few localized cysts in the left periventricular white matter. He went on to develop a mild asymmetrical diplegia, which improved with time, and a marked squint which eventually required surgery.

(a) The aEEG was started when the ultrasound abnormalities were first seen on day 5. The top trace shows a discontinuous burst-suppression pattern with fluctuations in the minimum amplitude that could represent a seizure pattern. Frequent arousals and caregiving could give the same aEEG pattern. Because of the clinical behavior with hiccups, in combination with the suspected seizure activity, phenobarbitone (phenob) was given. Twenty minutes after the phenobarbitone administration, a few clearly seizure-suspected changes appeared in the aEEG (at asterisk). In the middle part of the recording, a few suspected single seizures (asterisks) can be seen. A seizure pattern (asterisks), once again, became more clear in the lower trace and was stopped by a second dose of clonazepam (clona).

(b) Cranial ultrasound (parasagittal view) showing an area of increased echogenicity in the periventricular parietal white matter which evolved into localized cystic lesions (arrow) 5 weeks later.

(c) MRI, coronal slice, FLAIR (fluid attenuated inversion recovery) sequence (c) was performed at 2 years of age, and shows bilateral gliotic changes in the periventricular white matter.

The development of PVL in preterm infants is often accompanied by abnormal electrocortical background and epileptic seizure activity which is often subtle or subclinical

PVL in a preterm infant with surgical problems

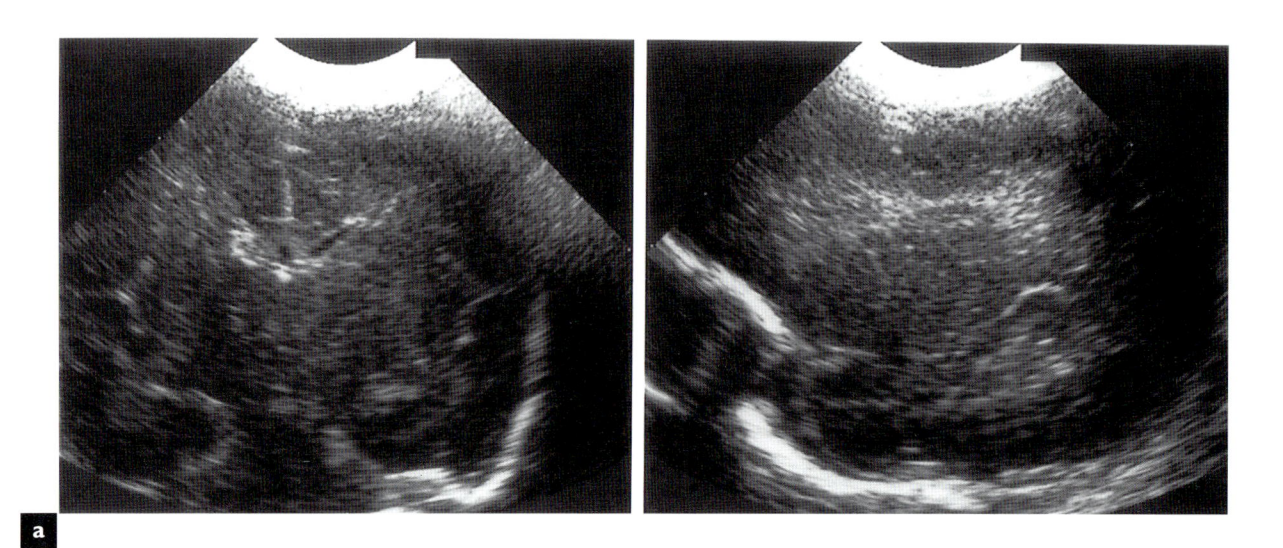

Figure 5.11 This female infant was born at 31 weeks' gestation by Cesarean section because of maternal pre-eclampsia. She was initially well and was not ventilated. However, at 5 days she suddenly deteriorated with clinical signs of necrotizing enterocolitis and was then referred to the regional NICU. On admission she had a loud cardiac murmur suggestive of a hemodynamic significant persistent ductus arteriosus. The ductus was closed surgically and she was stabilized before abdominal surgery was performed. The whole colon was resected and she had an ileostoma. During the 24 h following surgery for the necrotizing enterocolitis her clinical condition deteriorated. There were major problems in maintaining adequate arterial blood pressure. As her neurological condition also worsened intensive care treatment was withdrawn.

(a) Cranial ultrasound (coronal and parasagittal views) performed over the days only showed a germinal layer hemorrhage on the right, and mild patchy flaring in the periventricular white matter.

(b) The aEEG was started on day 5 following surgery for the persistent ductus arteriosus. The initial aEEG showed a burst-suppression background without sleep–wake cycling. The background pattern and the burst density cannot be considered as clearly abnormal for the gestational age in view of the analgesia and the previous anesthesia. However, on the second trace, recurrent epileptic seizures with a duration of 2–3 min emerged. The transient rise in the background activity in the middle part of the tracing, of 50-min duration, is probably not due to seizure activity but could be related to movement artefacts or pressure on the aEEG electrodes. Phenobarbitone (phenob) was given at the end of this tracing.

The seizure pattern ceased for several hours after phenobarbitone (third tracing). The aEEG background became more depressed with a sparse burst-suppression pattern, which was interrupted by three short suspected seizures on the second half of the tracing. There is also a drift in the baseline which is difficult to explain, but sometimes occurs in the aEEG when the electrocortical background is severely depressed. The source of this extremely low-voltage baseline activity could be extracranial. Since the amplitude is extremely low, a few microvolts, it is likely that it will not show in a standard EEG even if the origin is cerebral. The seizures recurred, and first lidocaine (lido) and then clonazepam (clona) were administered (fourth trace). Again the aEEG background became extremely low in amplitude, mainly inactive, before a sparse burst-suppression pattern reappeared (fifth tracing).

The bottom trace shows recurrence of a suspected seizure pattern with short seizure activity which lasts most of the tracing, and three more evident seizures on the second half. During the whole recording this infant received morphine because of the two surgical procedures. She had only one clinical seizure (asterisk) on the fourth tracing, and once a drop in saturation (sa) that was suspected to be a subtle seizure.

This recording shows the use of the aEEG following surgical procedures in severely ill preterm infants. It also shows that electrocortical background abnormalities can precede the appearance of ultrasound abnormalities in showing areas of periventricular ischemia

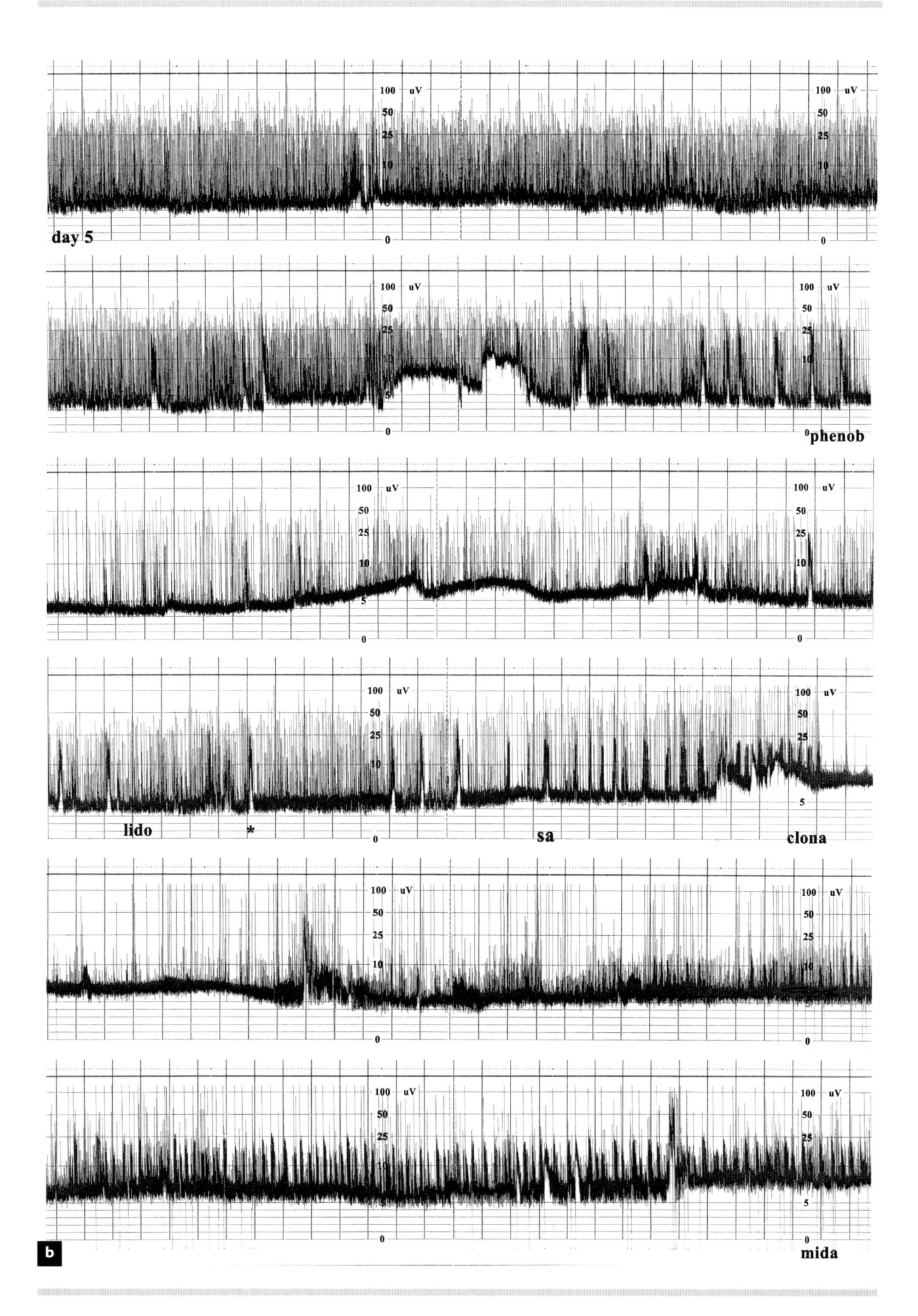

PVL and recurrent seizures

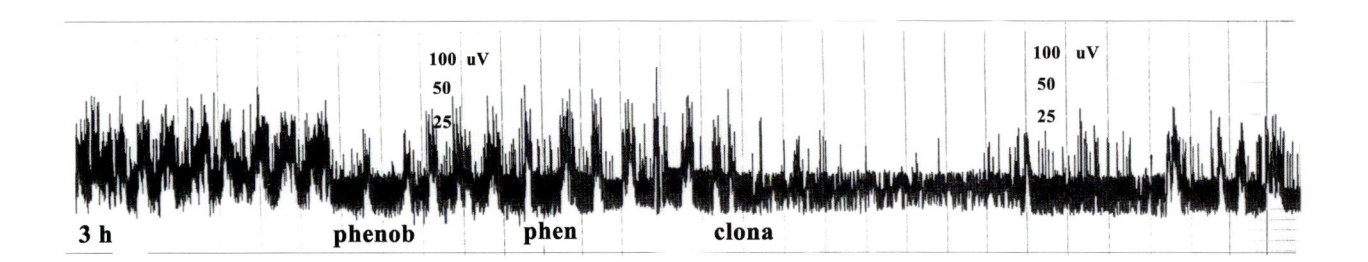

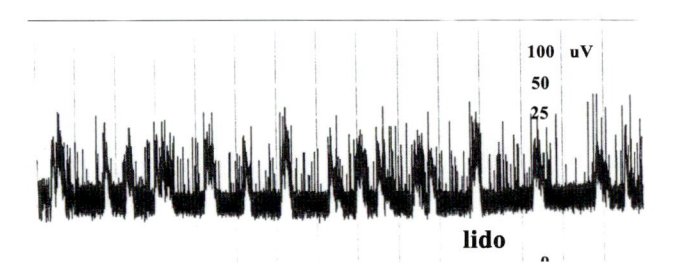

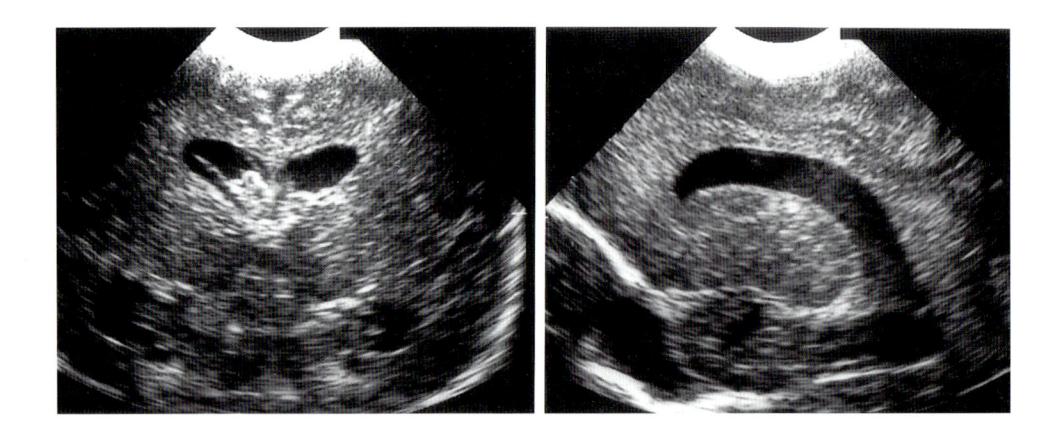

Figure 5.12 *opposite*   This preterm male infant was part of a monozygous twin pregnancy complicated by twin–twin transfusion syndrome (TTTS). The twins were delivered by Cesarean section at 31 weeks' gestation. This twin was the recipient with initial blood hemoglobin of 13 mmol/l. His birth weight was 2450 g and he was edematous and had abdominal distension due to ascites. His Apgar scores were 4 and 8, at 1 and 5 min, respectively. The umbilical artery pH was 6.98 and the base excess –17 mmol/l, and the first arterial lactate level was 19 mmol/l. He was intubated and ventilated and required high-frequency ventilation to be well oxygenated. Clinical seizures developed shortly following admission.

A cranial ultrasound scan was performed on admission and showed a small GMH–IVH mild ventricular dilatation with fresh blood in the lateral ventricles, and ischemic changes in the periventricular white matter. Because of anticipated very poor neurological prognosis, intensive care treatment was withdrawn. A postmortem examination confirmed extensive ischemic changes in liver, kidneys, heart and brain.

On admission, at 3 h of age, the aEEG was started and showed recurrent epileptic seizures ('saw-tooth' pattern) on a low-voltage background. A short effect on the seizure pattern was seen following phenobarbitone (phenob), with increased inter-ictal interval and a reduction in seizure amplitude, but the seizure pattern recurred. Phenytoin (phen) had no effect on the seizures but clonazepam (clona) seemed to interrupt the seizure pattern for more than an hour. The background activity after clonazepam (clona) became almost inactive, but it is possible that an extremely low-voltage seizure activity was still present during this period. The seizures pattern recurred with low-amplitude seizures lasting for 3–5 min and with 5–15-min intervals. Lidocaine (lido) was also administered but had no effect on the seizure pattern.

The clinical symptoms, cranial ultrasound and aEEG findings with recurrent seizure activity and depressed background are all evidence of severe congenital brain injury in this preterm infant

PVL in a preterm infant with gastroschisis and trisomy 21

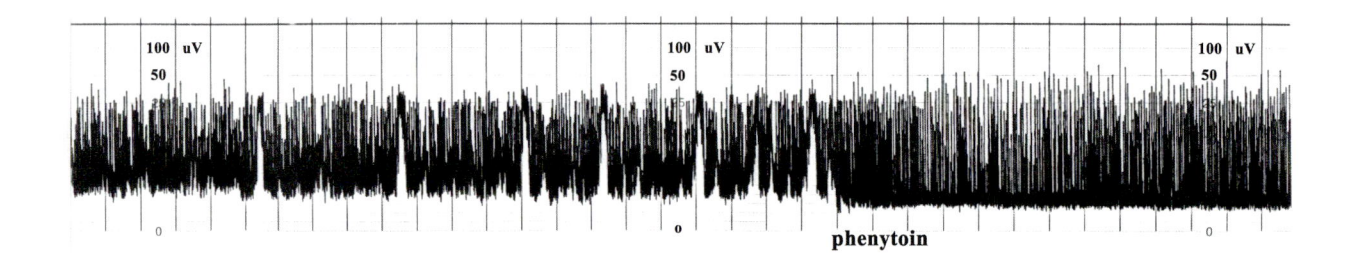

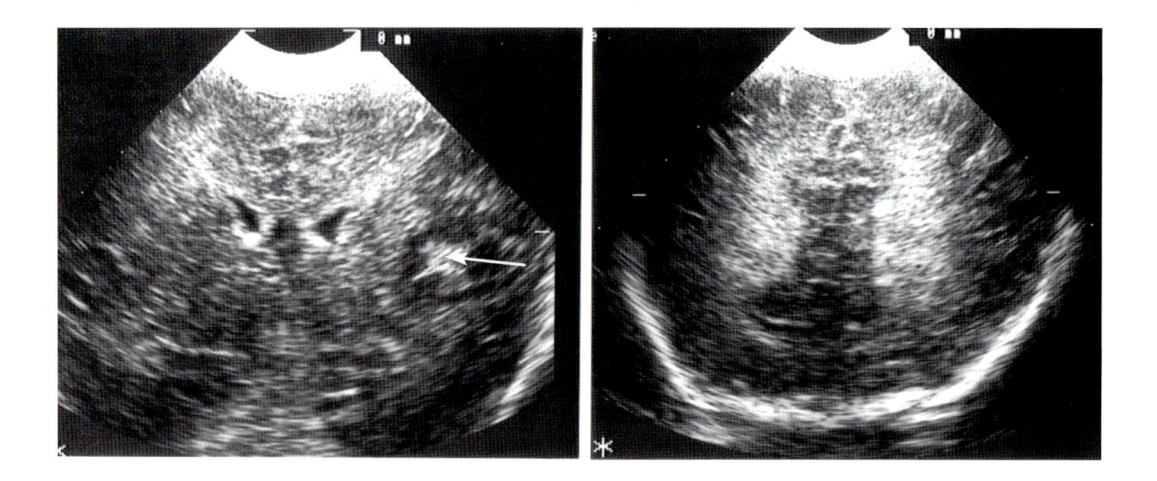

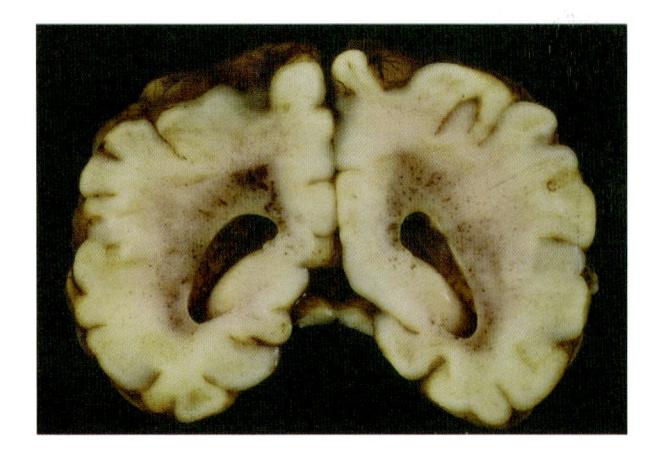
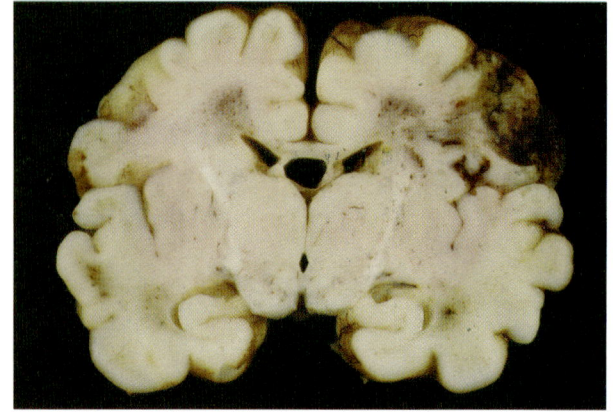

Figure 5.13 *opposite*   This female infant with a gestational age of 34 weeks and trisomy 21 was admitted for surgery due to gastroschisis. A routine cranial ultrasound scan was performed as part of the examination on admission. She had no clinical seizures. A middle cerebral artery infarct was seen in the left hemisphere (arrow) as well as extensive periventricular echodensities.

Because of the ultrasound findings, the aEEG was started before the planned surgery. The aEEG background was discontinuous and showed a burst-suppression background with repetitive electrographic seizures. The seven clear seizures can be identified as transient increases in the minimum amplitude of 2–3-min duration. Following administration of phenytoin, the electrographic seizures stopped and a burst-suppression background pattern remained. Because of the associated severe cerebral lesions it was finally decided not to continue intensive care treatment.

The postmortem examination confirmed the cerebral changes seen using ultrasonography. Courtesy of Dr P. Nikkels, Wilhelmina Children's Hospital, Utrecht, The Netherlands

6

Intracranial hemorrhage and aEEG

This chapter discusses aEEG features in preterm infants with GMH–IVH and intracranial hemorrhage (ICH) in full-term infants.

Electrocortical background abnormalities are common in preterm infants with GMH–IVH, and can precede cranial ultrasound abnormalities[61,63]. The early acute EEG changes, when the hemorrhage is developing, are characterized by depressed background activity and the presence of epileptic seizure activity. The degree of EEG and aEEG background depression is directly related to the size of the GMH–IVH[39,61–63,123,126,127]. This correlation has also been confirmed in postmortem studies[121]. Usually, the EEG background depression recovers within 1–2 weeks[63]. In preterm infants with a large GMH–IVH, the rate of recovery is predictive of later neurological outcome[123].

Epileptic seizure activity, often entirely subclinical or with only subtle clinical manifestations, is common during the development of GMH–IVH[39,61–63,126]. In a cohort of premature infants (mean gestational age 28 weeks) who had an aEEG during their first days of life, epileptic seizure activity was detected in two-thirds of the infants who developed GMH–IVH[63]. In a study including slightly more immature infants (mean gestational age 26 weeks) who had an aEEG during their first week of life, epileptic seizure activity was present in 75% of the infants who developed GMH–IVH[39]. The epileptic seizure activity that is associated with GMH–IVH is usually present only during the first days of life, when the hemorrhage is developing. The impact of the seizures on brain function, and their relation to later outcome, is not known. However, in infants with a large IVH, repetitive epileptic seizure activity did not seem to be associated with poor outcome[123].

Early prediction of neurological outcome from an aEEG is more uncertain in preterm infants than in full-term asphyxiated infants, since the degree of prematurity and other related (non-neurological) problems, e.g. chronic lung disease, also influence outcome. However, there is a correlation between aEEG background and degree of GMH–IVH, and the early electrocortical background activity subsequently also contains predictive information in preterm infants.

In preterm infants with grade III–IV GMH–IVH, graded according to Papile and colleagues[133], the maximum number of aEEG bursts/h during the first 48 h of life were shown to be predictive of later outcome. This is in accordance with experimental findings during recovery from hypoxia–ischemia in piglets, where burst occurrence and burst rate were predictive of outcome[122]. Preterm infants with large IVH and a higher burst rate than 130 bursts/h had a 70–80% chance of surviving in full health or with a minor to moderate handicap, as compared to infants with lower burst density who were more likely to die or survive with a severe handicap[123]. However, the cut-off level at 130 cannot be directly used, since the study was retrospective and most infants received phenobarbitone. The presence of sleep–wake cycling towards the end of the first week was also predictive of a relatively good outcome[123]. Sleep–wake cycling in aEEG is also associated with good outcome in extremely preterm infants with smaller or no GMH–IVH[39,40].

The following aEEG changes are associated with development of GMH–IVH in preterm infants:

- Increased discontinuity – characterized by increased interburst interval (lower burst density) and/or decreased amplitude (voltage) during interburst intervals;

- Lack of reactivity to care procedures;

- Lack of sleep–wake cycling;

- Presence of epileptic seizure activity;

- The aEEG abnormalities usually recover in 1–2 weeks.

In full-term infants, an ICH is often associated with birth trauma, coagulopathies or vascular malformations. There are no specific aEEG findings associated with ICH in full-term infants. As for preterm infants with GMH–IVH, ICH in full-term infants is often accompanied by temporary electrocortical depression and epileptic seizure activity. The degree of background abnormality is usually related to the severity of the brain injury.

Small and large GMH–IVH

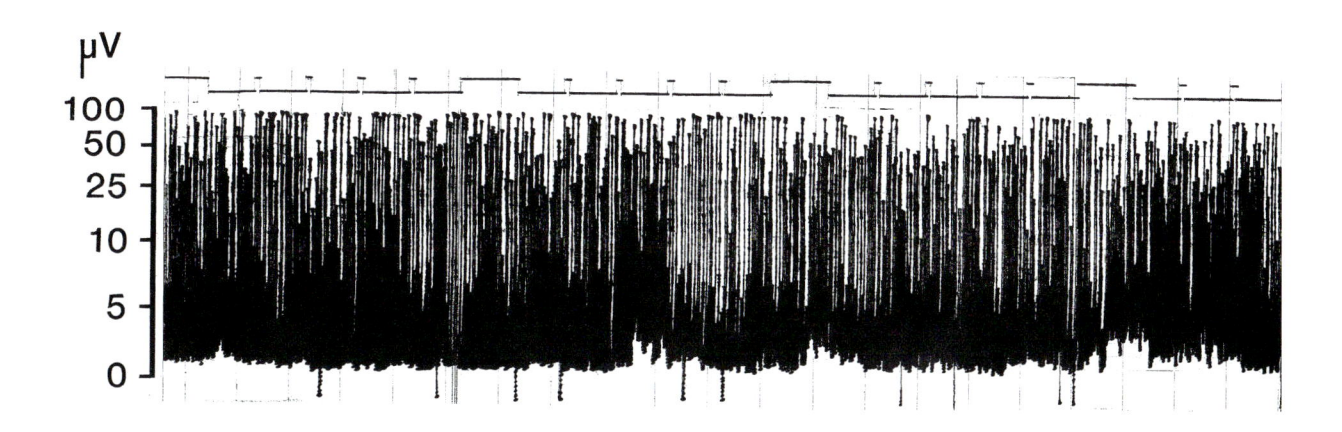

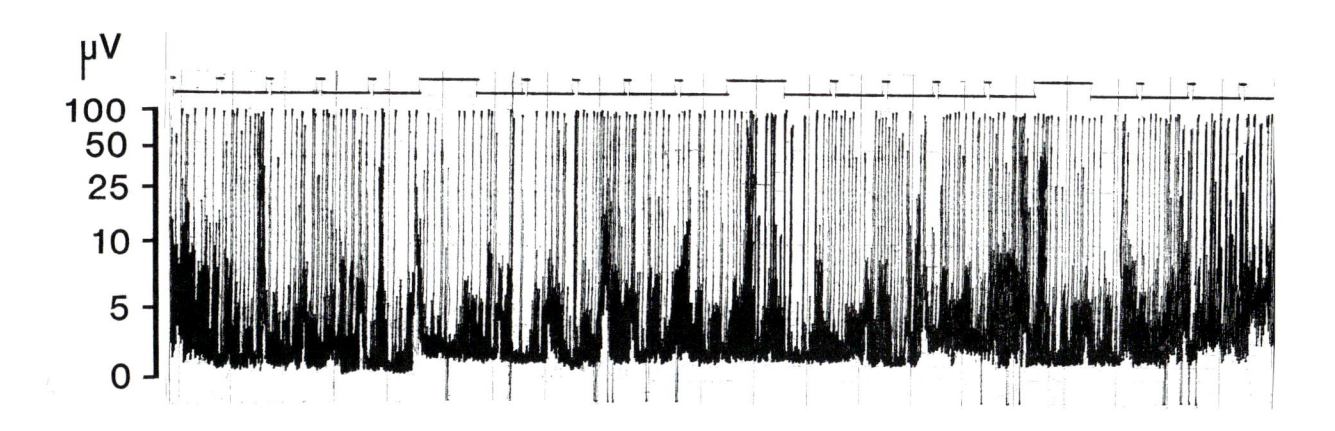

Figure 6.1 These two tracings illustrate the differences in aEEG background activity between infants with a small GMH–IVH versus a large hemorrhage. The upper tracing was recorded when this infant of 29 weeks' gestation had an IVH grade I, and the lower trace when the hemorrhage had developed to an IVH grade IV. The increased depression is represented by a decrease in burst density. The upper tracing shows some variability of the minimum amplitude but no sleep–wake cycling, which is also sometimes present in infants with large hemorrhages and is associated with good outcome. In the lower tracing some suspected seizure activity is also present

Infant with small GMH–IVH but poor outcome

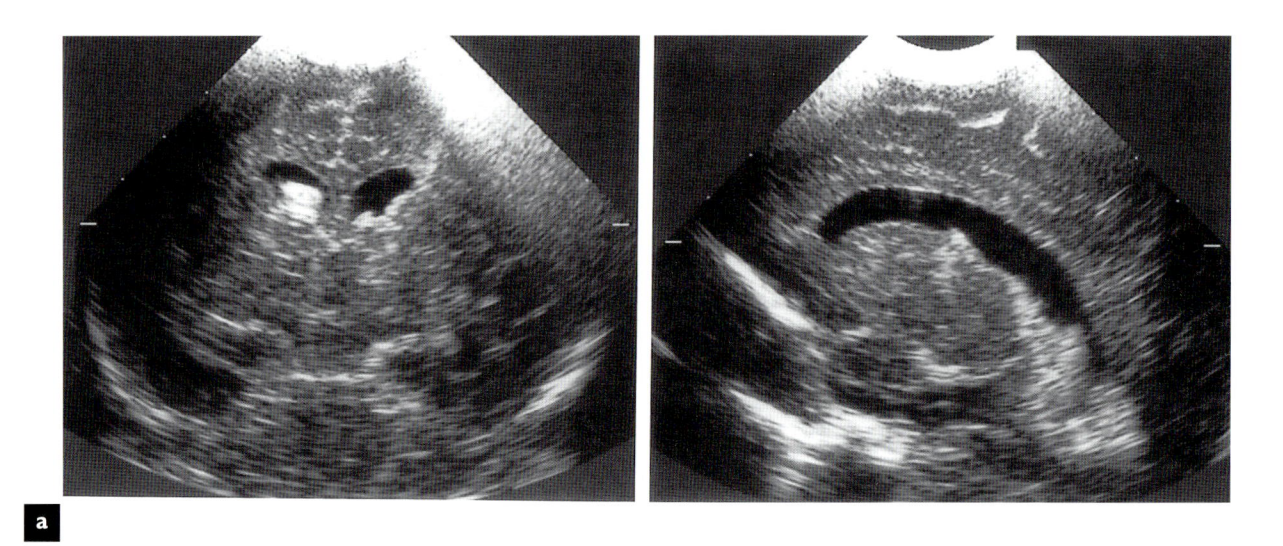

a

Figure 6.2 *above and opposite* This female infant was born by Cesarean section after 31 weeks' gestation, as there were indications of intrauterine infection. The birth weight was 1950 g. Her Apgar scores were 3 at 1 min, and 7 at 5 min. She developed grunting and required increasing amounts of oxygen before she was intubated. She was then transferred to the regional NICU. She had signs of infection with low platelets (76×10^9/l) and white cell counts (6.2×10^9/l). On arrival she was in poor condition with pH 6.98, $PaCO_2$ 104 mmHg, base excess –9 mmol/l and hemoglobin 6.1 mmol/l. An acute chest X-ray examination showed a tension pneumothorax, which was evacuated. During this period the infant suffered severe hypoxia and she also required cardiac massage and intratracheal adrenaline. After this event she developed pulmonary hypertension but responded to tolazoline infusion. Cardiac ultrasound showed poor contractility of the left ventricle, and she needed inotropic support with high doses of dopamine and dobutamine to maintain adequate blood pressure.

(a) The ultrasound scan showed a small GMH–IVH on the right side, which filled less than 50% of the lateral ventricles, and there was no increase in periventricular echogenicity. She deteriorated in spite of the intensive care treatment, which was withdrawn on day 5. Permission for a postmortem examination was not obtained.

(b) The aEEG was started several hours after the resuscitation. From the first aEEG a high-amplitude seizure pattern was already present which developed into a typical 'saw-tooth' pattern, corresponding to status epilepticus for several hours (two upper traces). There was no effect from a loading dose of clonazepam (second trace), but the seizure activity was temporarily stopped by phenytoin (third trace).

After the phenytoin, a burst-suppression background pattern was present for some hours before the seizure pattern recurred on a somewhat more discontinuous and lower-amplitude background than initially. Treatment with lidocaine finally stopped the seizure pattern (fourth trace).

The following aEEG (two lower traces) shows a burst-suppression pattern with low burst density, corresponding to one burst every 1–3 min.

This case shows that valuable additional information can be obtained from aEEG monitoring following a period with severe clinical deterioration. The cranial ultrasound diagnosis is not always sufficient to evaluate the possible brain injury. The etiology of the severe seizure activity in this infant was most likely severe hypoxic–ischemic brain injury

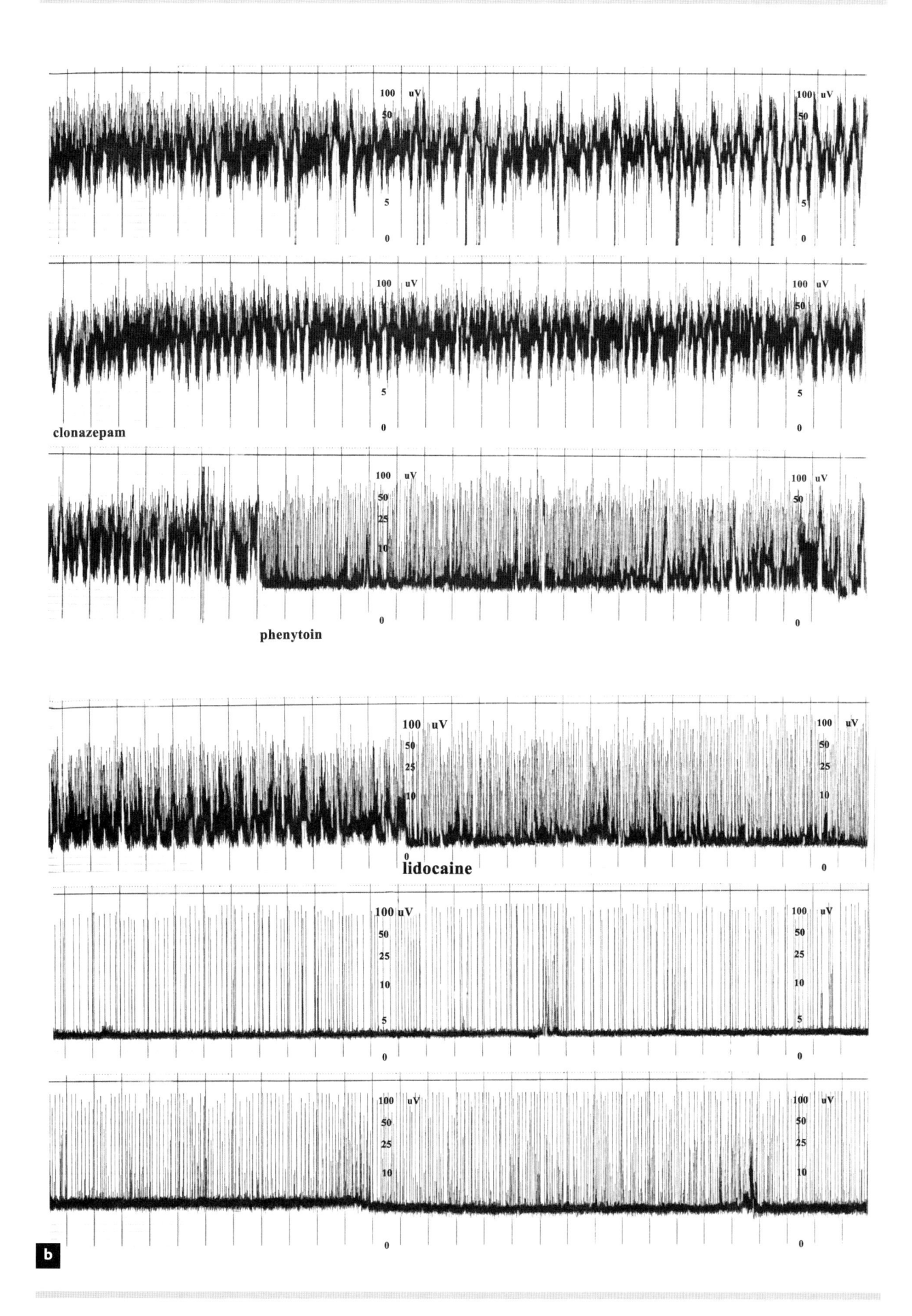

clonazepam

phenytoin

lidocaine

b

Infant with bilateral grade III hemorrhages but good outcome

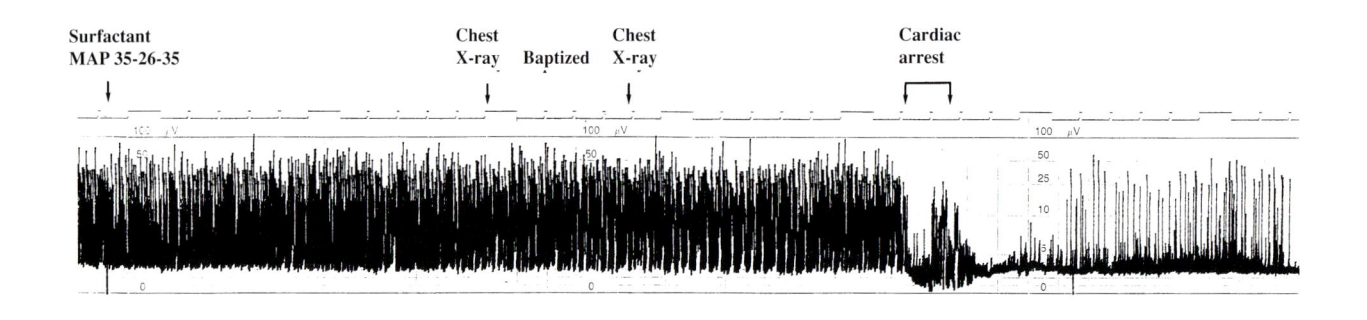

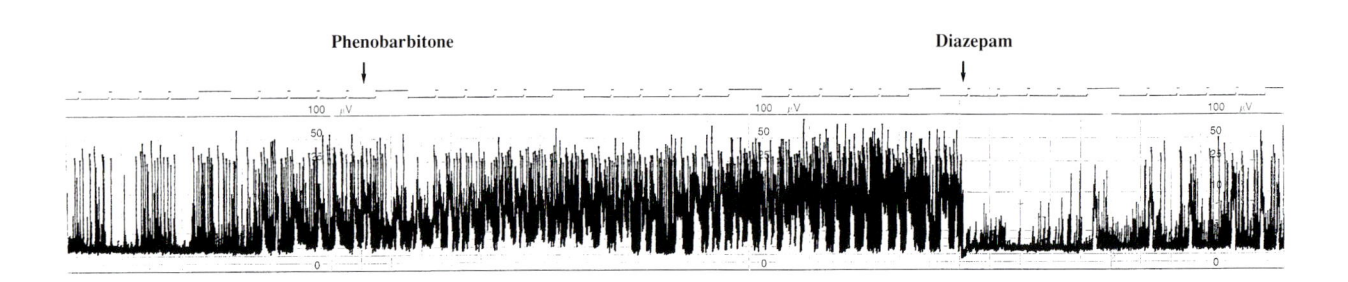

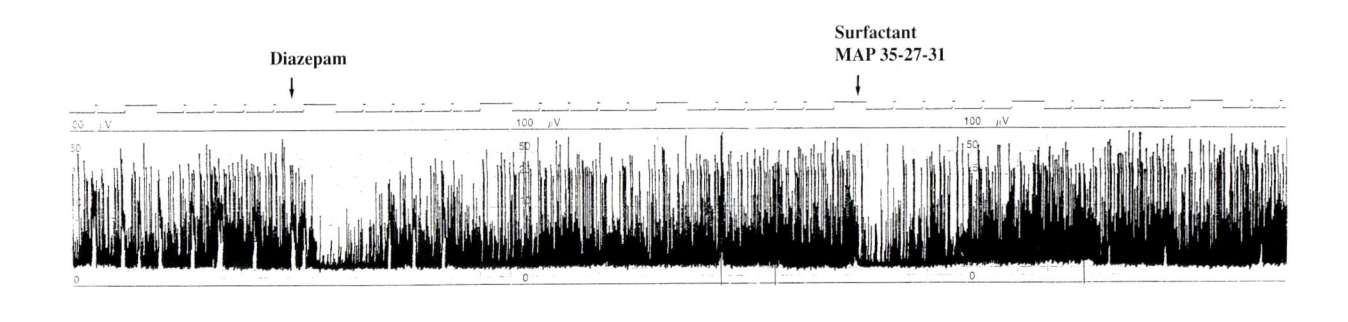

Age 4 days

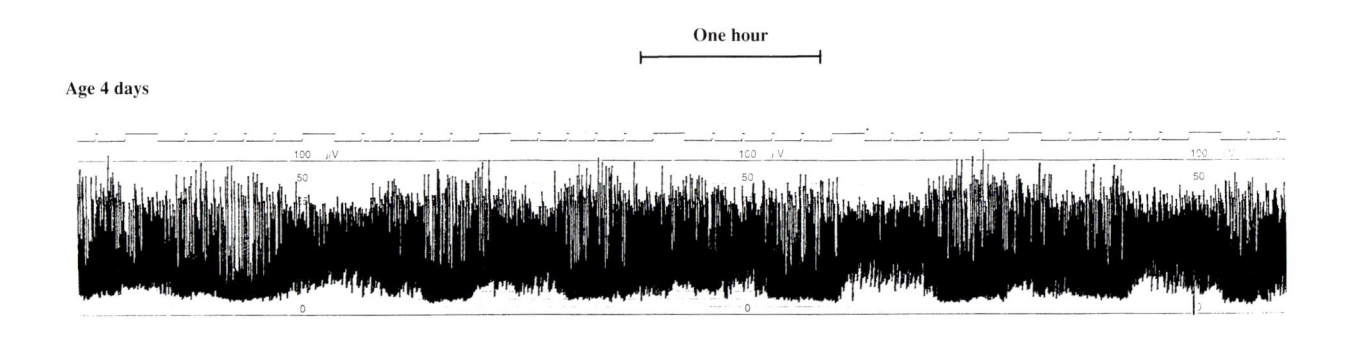

Figure 6.3 *opposite*   This male infant was born by emergency Cesarean section due to placental abruption at 30 weeks' gestation. He developed severe respiratory distress syndrome with recurrent bilateral pneumothoraces. On the 2nd day of life he developed cardiac arrest and was resuscitated (see below). He also developed bilateral GMH–IVH grade III. However, he survived and was normal at follow-up at 8 years of age.

The three upper aEEG traces constitute a continuous 20-h recording from days 2–3. The lowest trace was recorded on the infant's 4th day of life. Every trace corresponds to almost 7 h. The initial aEEG background was discontinuous and burst-suppression-like. In the beginning of the recording he was given surfactant, which resulted in a transient drop in mean arterial blood pressure but no effect on the aEEG. A 'saw-tooth' pattern, corresponding with repetitive epileptic seizure activity evolved but he had no clinical fits. He was in a critical condition and was baptised between the two X-ray examinations, and $1^1/_2$ hours later he developed cardiac arrest (upper trace). During resuscitation the aEEG became inactive and only movement artefacts were recorded during the following 40 min when he received cardiopulmonary resuscitation.

Cerebral activity then returned with a sparse burst-suppression pattern, which changed into a new 'saw-tooth' pattern with subclinical seizure activity (second trace). Diazepam abolished the seizure activity and the background activity was flat during the following hour. The epileptic seizure activity recurred but less frequently than before (seizure intervals 10–20 min). A second dose of diazepam was given, and three short seizures can be seen after this (third trace).

Another dose of surfactant was also given and this time resulted in a 'typical' response with transient aEEG depression for 10–20 min (third trace).

The bottom trace from day 4 shows periods with continuous activity and a cyclical pattern resembling sleep–wake cycling.

This example shows several events that can occur during neonatal intensive care in a critically ill infant. The rapid normalization of the aEEG background was predictive of a good outcome in spite of the previous severe aEEG abnormalities and the bilateral GMH–IVH

Bilateral grade IV hemorrhages with poor outcome

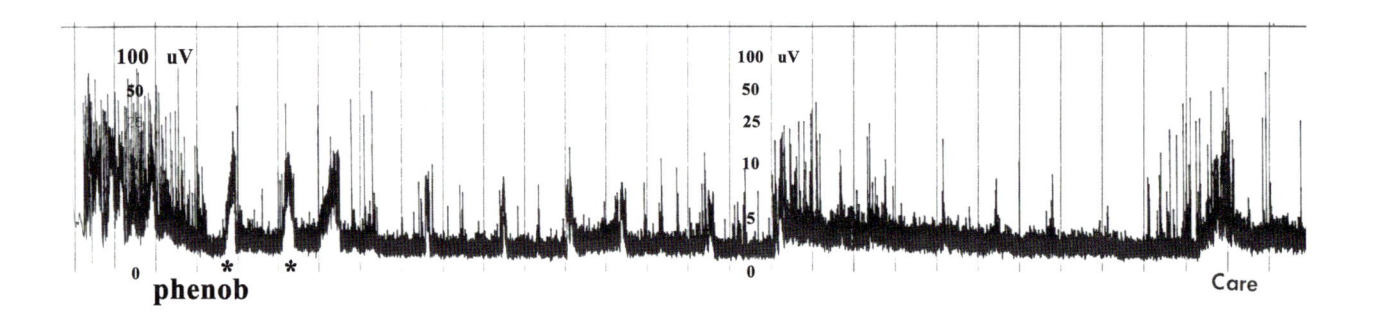

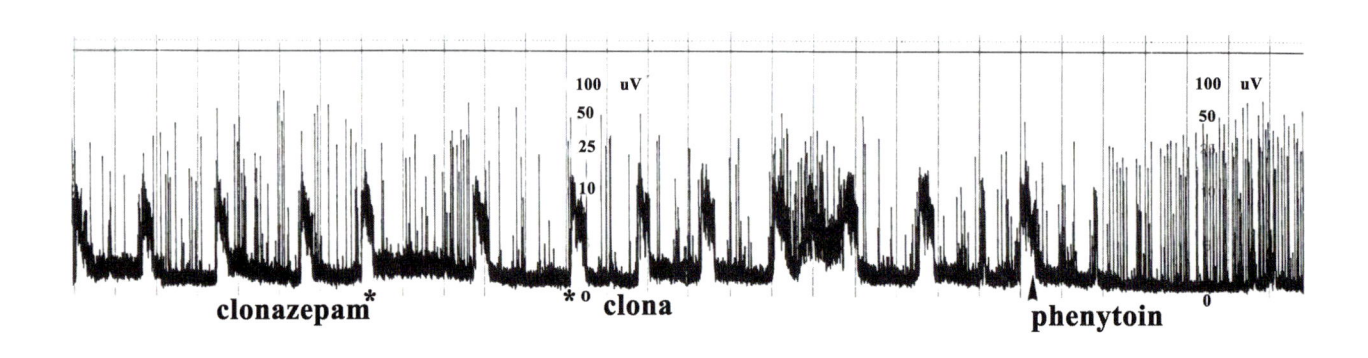

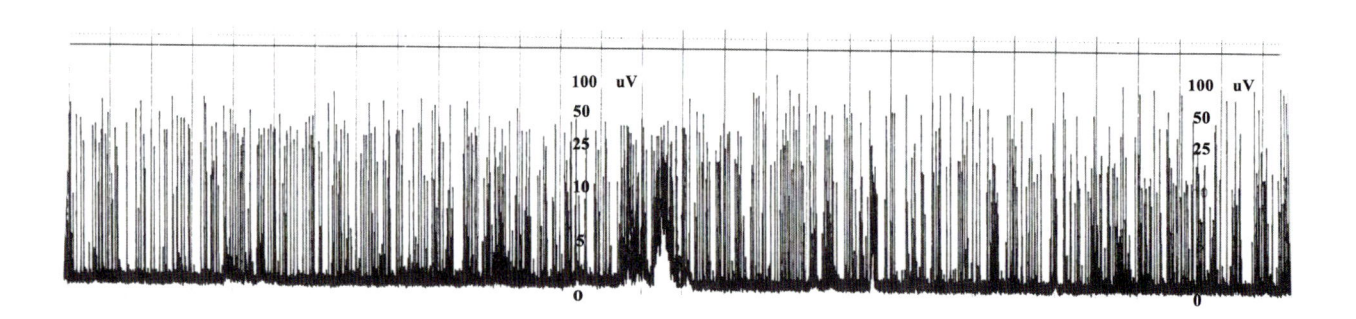

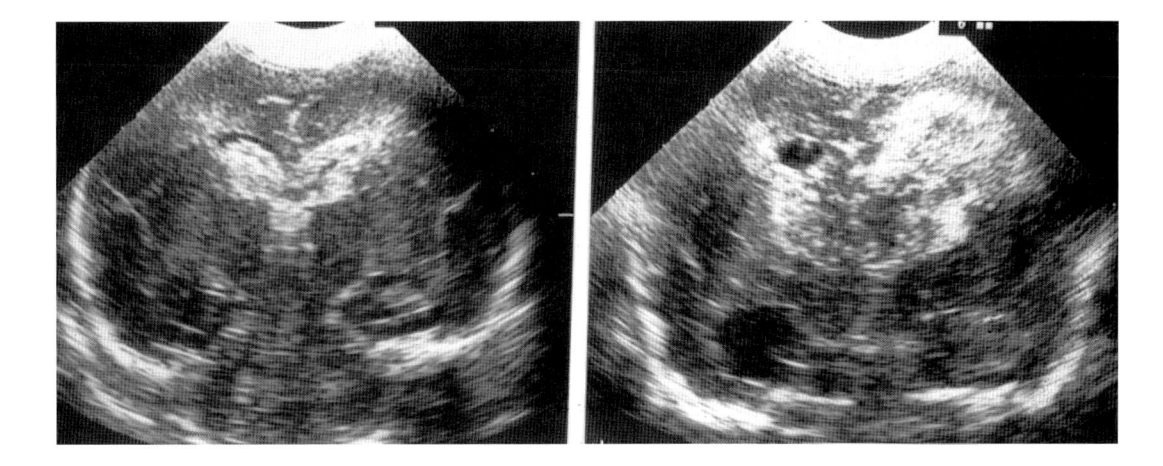

Figure 6.4 *opposite and above* This female twin was born at 29 weeks' gestation following 20 h of ruptured membranes. Her Apgar scores were 6 and 8 at 1 and 5 min, respectively. Her birth weight was 1540 g. Shortly after delivery she developed respiratory distress and was intubated and ventilated. She received antibiotics and the blood culture, as well as skin swabs, were positive for *Staphylococcus aureus*. On the 2nd day of life she had a sudden fall in her hemoglobin from 8.9 mmol/l to 4.6 mmol/l. The cranial ultrasound scan was normal on admission but progressesd from small bilateral intraventricular hemorrhages to bilateral parenchymal hemorrhages, most marked on the left, following the fall in hemoglobin.

The aEEG was started when the parenchymal hemorrhages were detected. The infant was then very irritable and also had clinical seizures (asterisks) with corresponding changes in the aEEG. The initial aEEG showed a burst-suppression pattern with short recurrent seizure activity. After phenobarbitone (phenob) administration, the background became severely depressed and mainly inactive. The epileptic seizure activity gradually stopped.

After some hours (middle trace), clinical and subclinical seizures recurred at 15–30-min intervals. Clonazepam (clona) did not affect the seizure activity, which was stopped when phenytoin was added.

The subsequent burst-suppression background pattern, with quite low burst density, was occasionally interrupted by a suspected seizure (third trace). The combination of the severe bilateral parenchymal hemorrhages, the epileptic seizure acitivity and the poor electrocortical background led to withdrawal of intensive care treatment.

The severely and continuously depressed aEEG background in this infant with bilateral parenchymal hemorrhages indicated poor outcome

Unilateral grade IVH with fair outcome

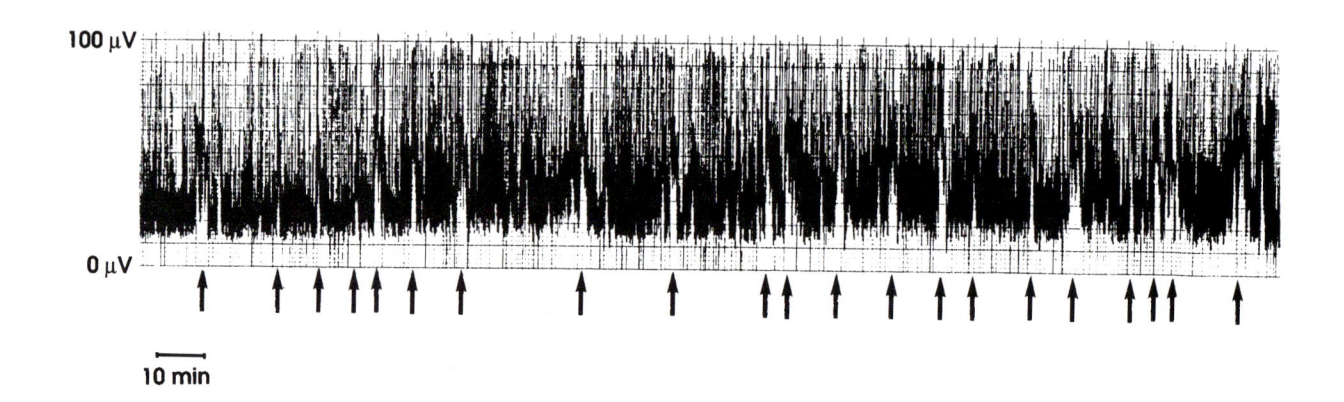

100 µV

0 µV

10 min

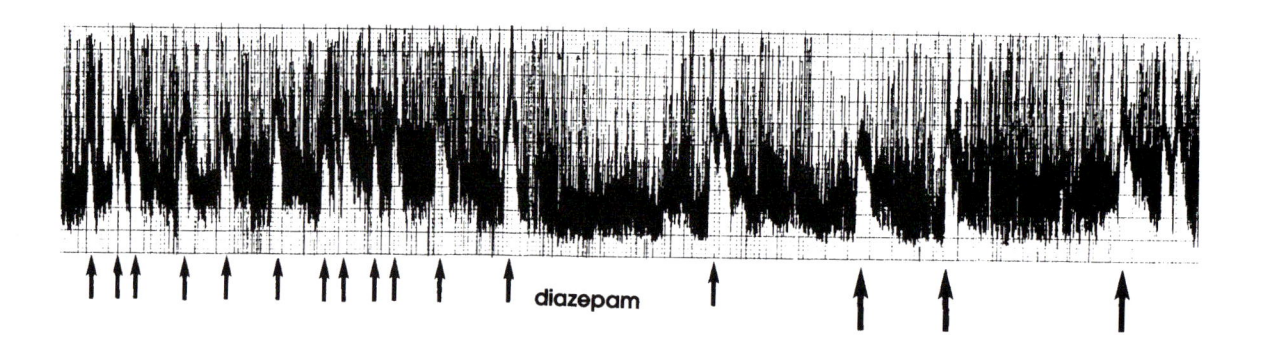

diazepam

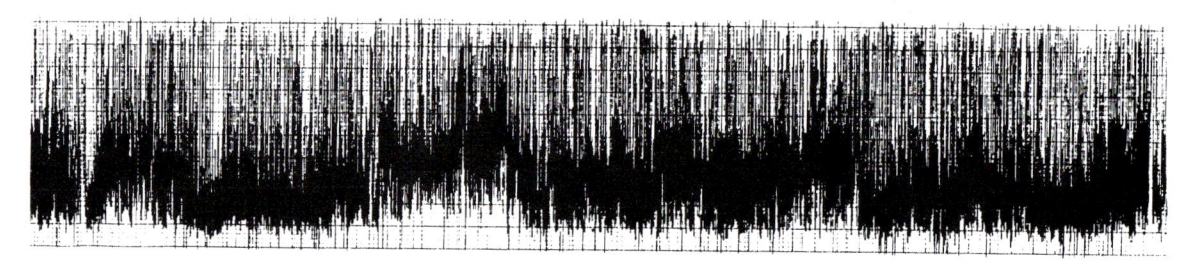

EEG

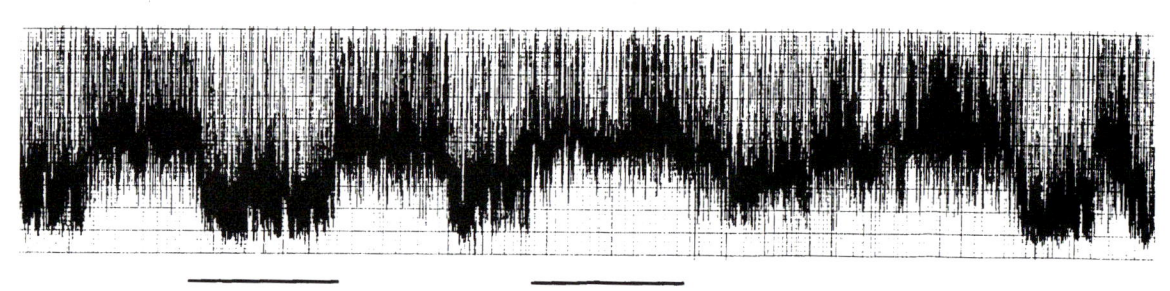

quiet sleep   awake / active sleep

Figure 6.5 *opposite*   This preterm female infant was born at 28 weeks' gestation after placental abruption. She needed mechanical ventilation for respiratory distress syndrome, and inotropic support for arterial hypotension. Cranial ultrasound enabled a diagnosis of a unilateral parenchymal hemorrhage, probably a venous infarction (IVH grade 4) on the 2nd day of life. She had aEEG as standard intensive care monitoring. She did not have any clinical seizures. On follow-up at 5 years of age this girl had developed moderate spastic diplegia, but she had a normal IQ and participated in normal preschool training.

The two upper traces show parts of her aEEG from days 2 and 3. The aEEG background was discontinuous and burst-suppression-like. Repeated electrographic seizure activity was present (arrows) and continued in spite of treatment with diazepam and phenobarbitone. The two lower traces were recorded on days 4 and 5. The background activity was still mainly discontinuous, as could be expected and adequate for her gestational age, but the epileptic seizure activity had ceased.

A standard EEG was performed, and confirmed the aEEG, and showed discontinuous background with no epileptic seizure activity. On day 4, an emerging cyclical pattern, resembling sleep–wake cycling, was becoming increasingly evident (lower two traces). The more discontinuous parts correspond with quiet-sleep periods, and the more continuous parts with wakefulness or active sleep.

The relatively fast normalization of the aEEG background, and development of sleep–wake cycling, is predictive of a relatively good outcome in spite of the severe hemorrhage. It can also be noted that the burst density during the first days was rather dense, a feature that is associated with fair outcome in preterm infants with large hemorrhages[123]

Full-term infant with an intracranial hemorrhage

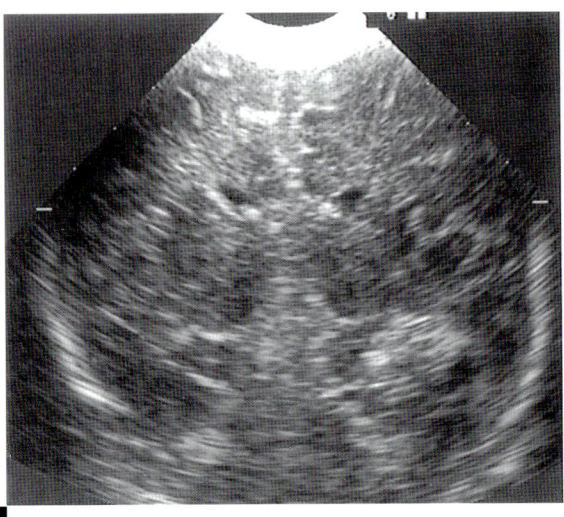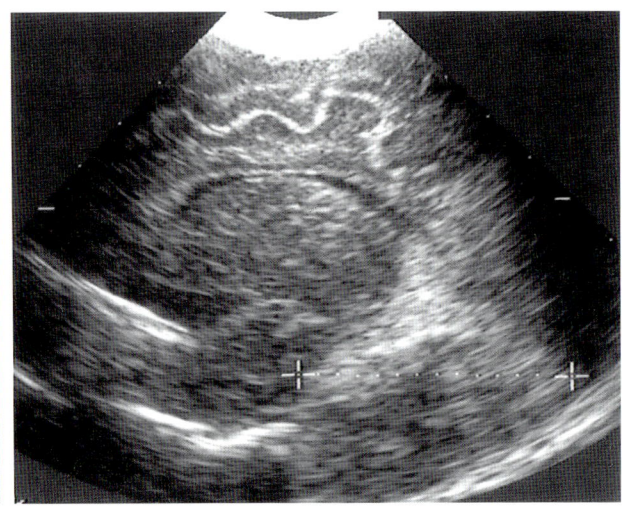

a

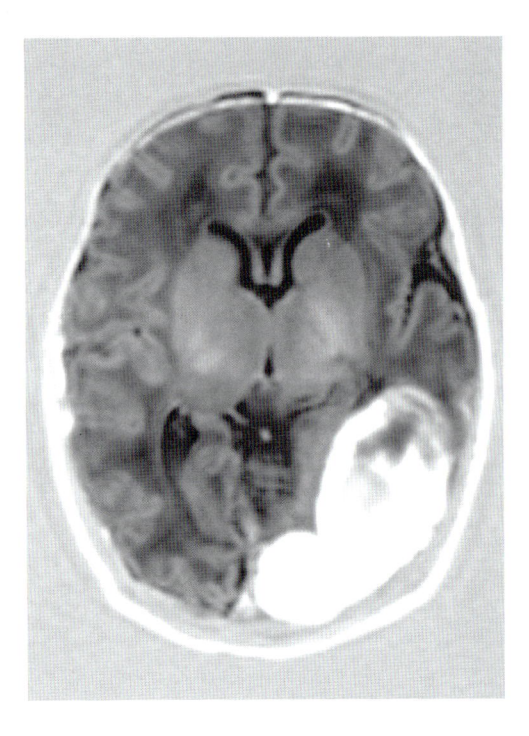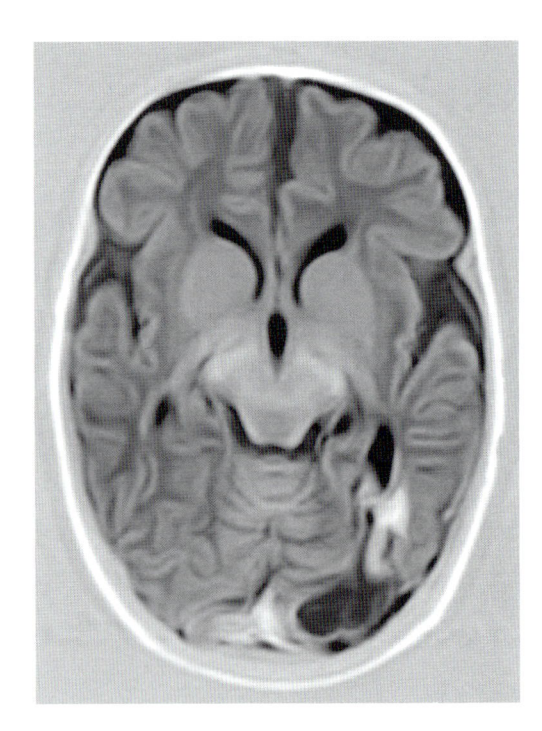

b

Figure 6.6 This female infant was born at 38 weeks' gestation and weighed 2540 g. The mother had been treated for hypertension. The amniotic fluid was meconium-stained and the delivery was precipitous, but she had a good start with Apgar scores 8 and 10 at 1 and 5 min, respectively. She appeared well enough to be admitted to the postnatal ward, but because of a first low blood glucose she was transferred to the special care baby unit. Within a few hours she developed repeated apneas and required mechanical ventilation, and was transferred to the NICU. Following admission, the blood glucose levels were normal.

(a) A cranial ultrasound scan (coronal and parasagittal views) showed a large area of increased echogenicity in the left parieto-occipital lobe.

(b) This was subsequently confirmed to be a large parenchymal hemorrhage on MRI which was performed during the first week and at 3 months, using the inversion recovery sequence, and shows the evolution from a large lobar hemorrhage to a relatively small area of cavitation. The infant recovered and the neurodevelopmental outcome at 18 months of age was within the normal range (developmental quotient 99)

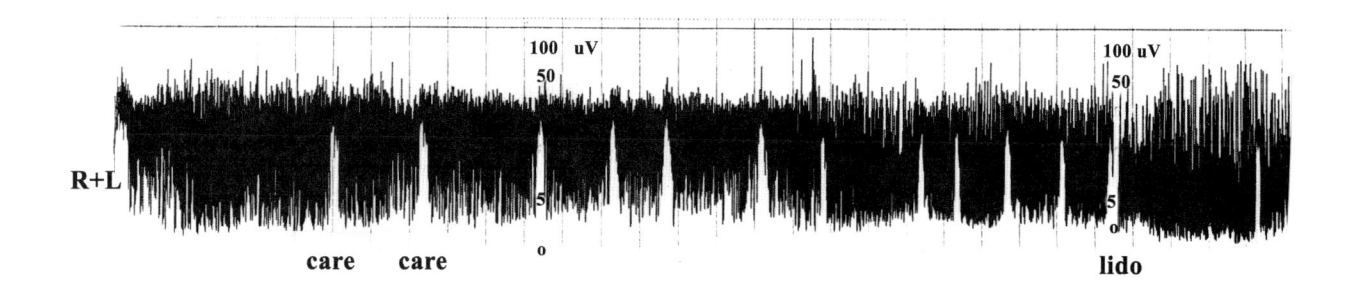

day 2

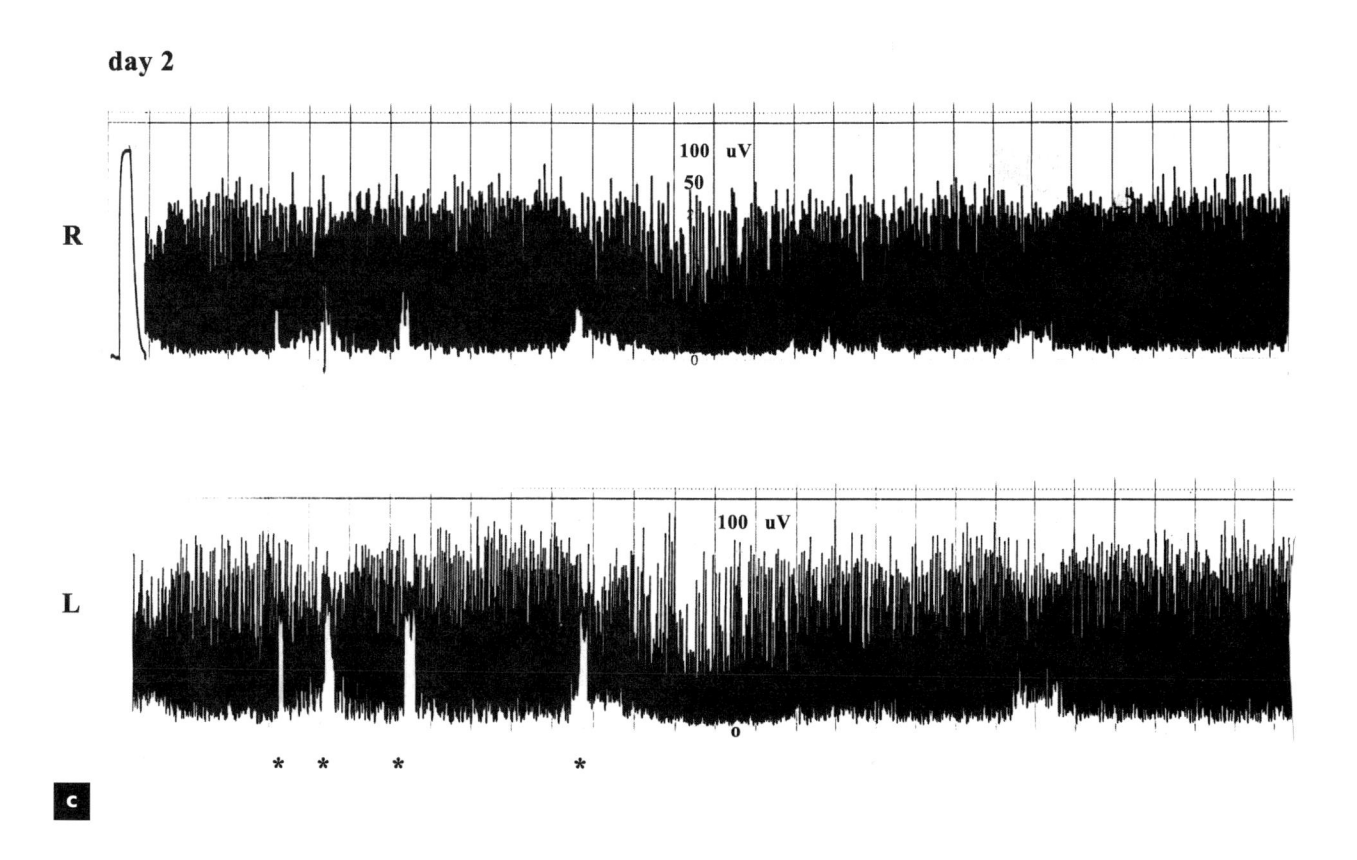

Figure 6.6 continued (c) Immediately following admission, aEEG monitoring was started. The background was discontinuous and suspected repeated seizure activity was seen as short transient increases in the minimum amplitude. The infant did not have any clinical seizures. Some of the suspected seizure activity was associated with handling of the infant. Since an EEG was not performed here, it is impossible to say whether the care procedures elicited seizure activity or if the arousal from handling just looked very similar to the suspected seizure activity. She was treated with phenobarbitone and midazolam for the suspected seizures. Lidocaine (lido) was added to the medication, in an attempt to stop the subclinical seizure activity (upper bilateral recording). After the lidocaine administration, two channels of aEEG – one from each hemisphere (F3–P3 and F4–P4) – were recorded (R, right; L, left). Following the lidocaine, four electrographic seizures (asterisks) were recorded with the seizure activity being more evident on the left side with the hemorrhage. No asymmetry was present in the general background activity which was depressed and showed a burst-suppression pattern with no sleep–wake cycling.

This example shows the utility of bilateral recordings in infants with unilateral lesions

Full-term infant with subtentorial hemorrhage

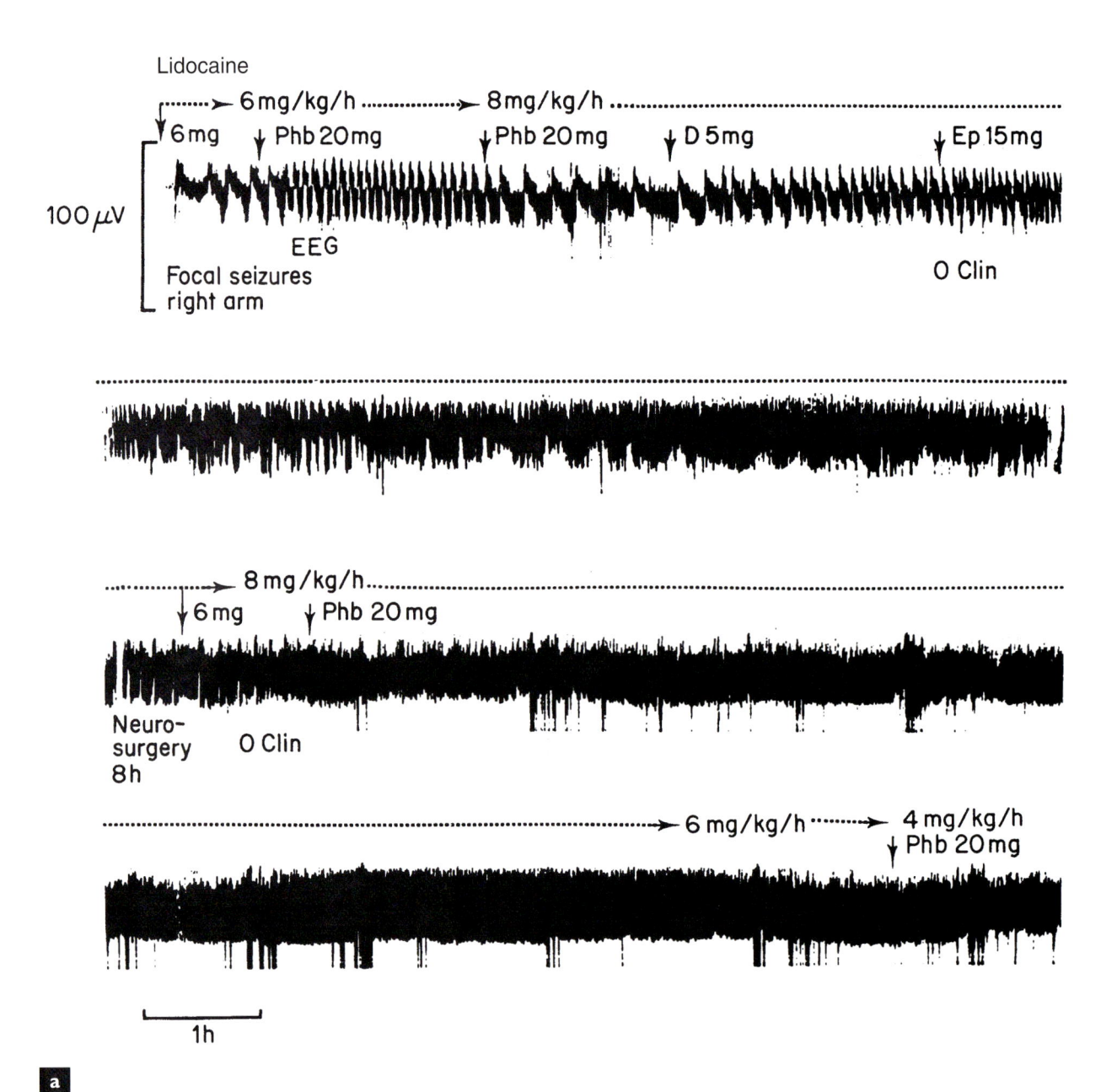

Figure 6.7   This full-term female infant was delivered using ventouse extraction because of a slowly progressing delivery. After birth, she needed manual ventilation for 5 min before she was stabilized. She was then admitted to the neonatal unit for observation. The Apgar scores were 3, 7 and 8 at 1, 5 and 10 min, respectively. Her birth weight was 4070 g. When she was 1¹/₂ h old, clonic seizures developed with right-sided predominance. Blood gases, blood glucose and blood hemoglobin were normal. A CT scan revealed a tentorial hemorrhage on the left side. She was subsequently referred to the regional NICU for treatment. On arrival she had focal clonic seizures involving the right arm.

(a) The aEEG was started soon after arrival. The repetitive focal seizures affecting the right arm corresponded with a high-amplitude 'saw-tooth' pattern in the aEEG. She was given a bolus and continuous intravenous infusion of lidocaine with no effect on the seizures

Full-term infant with subtentorial hemorrhage

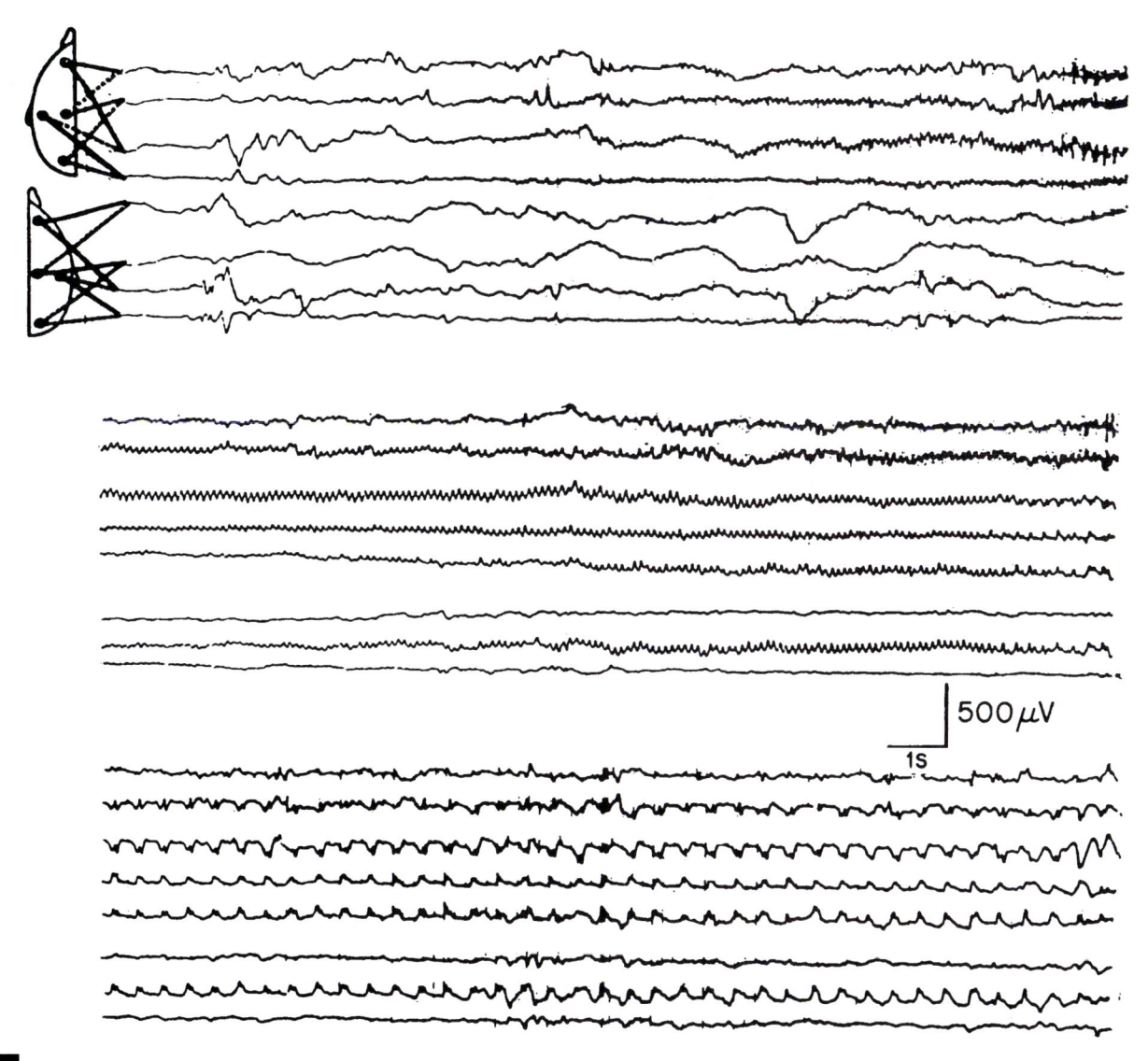

b

Figure 6.7 continued   (b) A standard EEG showed a typical seizure pattern with seizure onset on the left side with secondary generalization. After additional treatment with phenobarbitone (PhB), diazepam (D) and phenytoin (Ep) the clinical seizures ceased but repetitive electrographic seizure activity persisted for several hours (second aEEG trace). She went on to neurosurgery, and a subdural hematoma was evacuated. Immediately postoperatively there was a transient period with electrographic seizure activity. Anticonvulsive treatment was gradually withdrawn. The aEEG background was mainly discontinuous, although the infant did not have a burst-suppression pattern since the minimum amplitude (lower border) of the tracing is not zero but of relatively low amplitude. She gradually recovered and returned to the referral hospital. Reproduced from reference 134 with permission.

This example shows that epileptic seizure can be very intense in infants with intracranial hemorrhages. It also shows that clinical seizures may continue as subclinical seizure activity after antiepileptic treatment, and how the aEEG can be used for monitoring of the possible recurrence of seizure activity during withdrawal of antiepileptic treatment

7

aEEG and metabolic diseases, central nervous system infections and brain malformations

Hypoglycemia is a frequent cause of cerebral dysfunction in newborn infants. Most EEG findings associated with hypoglycemia and many of the rare metabolic diseases are non-specific. The degree of cerebral dysfunction is correlated with EEG background abnormalities and the presence of epileptiform and epileptic seizure activity. Early hypoglycemic EEG changes include an increase in lower EEG frequencies, which is impossible to detect with the aEEG, as shown in full-term infants with moderate hypoglycemia[135,136]. Severe hypoglycemia is associated with aEEG background depression and epileptic seizure activity as shown in the examples below and in Figure 1.4.

A burst-suppression EEG background is associated with some severe encephalopathies, such as non-ketotic hyperglycinemia, hemimegalencephaly and Ohtahara syndrome[137–140]. Other EEG findings, including asymmetries and epileptic seizure activity, may also be present. Some of the background EEG changes associated with these diseases can also be found in the aEEG, as seen in the examples below.

Pyridoxine-dependent seizures are quite rare but the incidence is probably underestimated[141]. The two examples below of infants with pyridoxine-responsive seizures are probably quite typical in their clinical presentation. They also show the different responses to pyridoxine administration that have been described[142]. Neither of these two infants had the standard EEG pattern, consisting of generalized bursts of 1–4 Hz sharp and slow activity, that has been described as typical for pyridoxine-dependent seizures[143,144].

When using aEEG monitoring in infants with metabolic brain dysfunction it is also important to record at least one standard EEG, since subtle electrocortical background changes are not possible to detect with the aEEG. The aEEG samples below cannot cover all rare metabolic diseases but show how the aEEG can be used to give continuous information on brain function and its development during the clinical course in these infants.

Cerebral symptoms due to central nervous system infections or brain malformations are not uncommon. As for metabolic brain dysfunction, the EEG abnormalities are usually non-specific and include changes in the background activity and presence of epileptic seizure activity. Such background changes are feasible to follow with aEEG monitoring as seen in the examples. As for the majority of patients with cerebral dysfunction at least one standard EEG should be performed. Changes in the EEG background, such as a multifocal periodic pattern which has been associated with neonatal herpes simplex meningoencephalitis, are not possible to detect with aEEG[145].

- Most electrocortical changes due to metabolic diseases, central nervous system infections or malformations are non-specific;

- The most common aEEG findings are changes in the general background activity and presence of epileptic seizure activity;

- A standard EEG should be recorded early in all infants with cerebral symptoms due to metabolic disturbances, including hypoglycemia, infections and cerebral malformations;

- Some rare diseases have specific EEG changes.

Postasphyctic hypoglycemia in a full-term infant

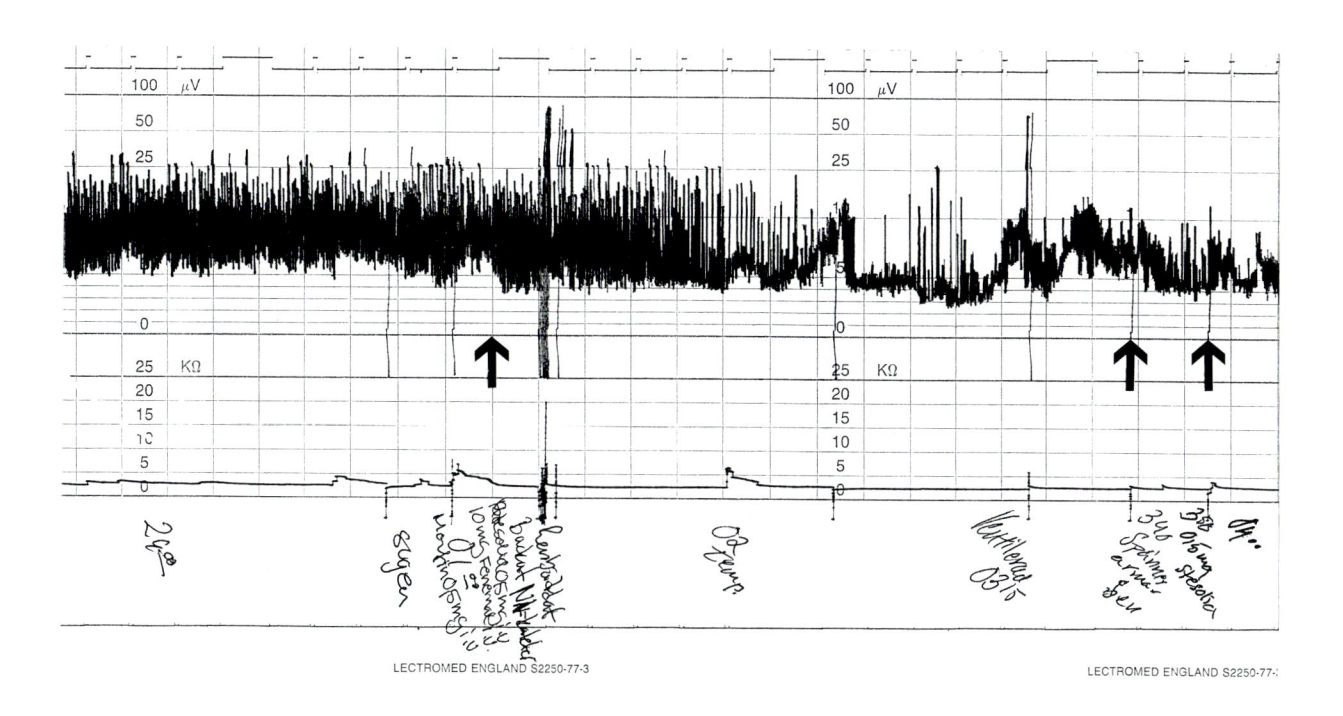

LECTROMED ENGLAND S2250-77-3

LECTROMED ENGLAND S2250-77-:

Figure 7.1   This full-term female infant was severely asphyxiated and needed mechanical ventilation. During the first postnatal hours she developed hypoglycemia, which was treated with a glucose infusion. In spite of this treatment the hypoglycemia deteriorated. Just before the beginning of the aEEG recording her blood glucose was only 0.96 mmol/l and during the recording the blood glucose deteriorated to zero. She survived with neurological handicap.

The infant was 6 h old at the beginning of this 4½-h sample from her aEEG recording. In the beginning, the aEEG background was continuous with normal voltage. This background pattern indicates good outcome after birth asphyxia. At the first arrow, she received 10 mg phenobarbitone, 0.5 mg diazepam and 0.5 mg morphine intravenously for sedation, and the aEEG background became slightly discontinuous (the weight of the tracing at the lower margin). After another hour the aEEG background deteriorated and became very depressed, almost inactive. At the second arrow she had a clinical seizure, and at the third arrow she received another dose of diazepam. The impedance recording is also shown. The impedance was mainly at 2–3 kΩ, which indicates the good quality of the recording. During care procedures, indicated by clinical notes below the tracings, the impedance transiently increased to 5–6 kΩ except for one occasion (after the first arrow) when it rose to 20 kΩ and the aEEG signal temporarily shut off.

It is possible that the hypoglycemia in this asphyxiated infant contributed to the development of the brain injury, since the initial aEEG was normal but deteriorated during the severe hypoglycemia

Hypoglycemia in a preterm infant with intrauterine growth restriction

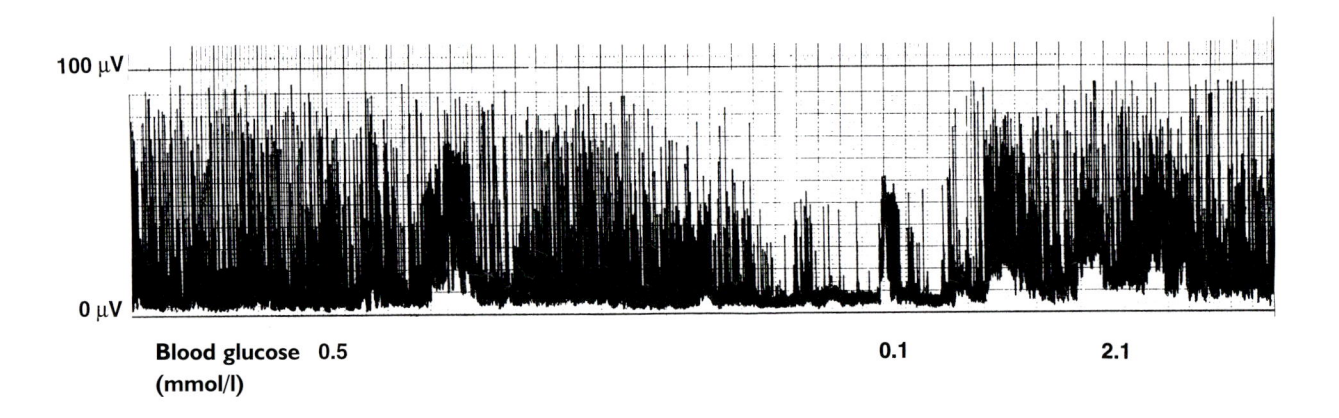

Figure 7.2 This female infant was born at 28 weeks' gestation after a pregnancy complicated by pre-eclampsia. She was growth restricted with a birth weight of 660 g, but she was vital at birth and her Apgar scores were 5, 9 and 9 at 1, 5 and 10 min, respectively. She acquired respiratory distress syndrome and a pulmonary hemorrhage. She received surfactant and also indomethacin for a symptomatic persistent ductus arteriosus. She also developed hypoglycemia. Initially, the hypoglycemia was accompanied by a few subtle seizures but 2 days later she also had a few clonic seizures. She survived and was discharged in good condition to a local hospital at 4 weeks. The cranial ultrasound before discharge showed two small periventricular cysts but was otherwise regarded as normal. Her long-term outcome is not known.

The aEEG (duration 4.3 h, paper speed 5 cm between vertical lines) was recorded on the infant's 3rd day of life. At that time she was supported by mechanical ventilation. The aEEG background was discontinuous and showed a burst-suppression pattern. The blood glucose values are given below the tracing. In the beginning of the recording the blood glucose level was 0.5 mmol/l, and she received betamethasone and an infusion with 20% glucose in order to increase the low blood glucose. In spite of this treatment, the blood glucose deteriorated further to 0.1 mmol/l, and, simultaneously, the aEEG became increasingly depressed. When the blood glucose was 0.1 mmol/l, the blood pressure became unstable, and she became tachycardic and was breathing against the ventilator. These symptoms could represent subtle seizure activity and fit with the simultaneous seizure-suspected transient rise in the aEEG. A bolus of glucose, and also diazepam were given. Cerebral activity recovered and the next blood glucose level was 2.1 mmol/l. The time-scale in this Figure is 5 min between the vertical lines.

This example shows how the cerebral activity in preterm infants can be affected by hypoglycemia, and also the improvement in the aEEG when the hypoglycemia was treated

Hypoglycemia in a full-term infant with necrotizing enterocolitis

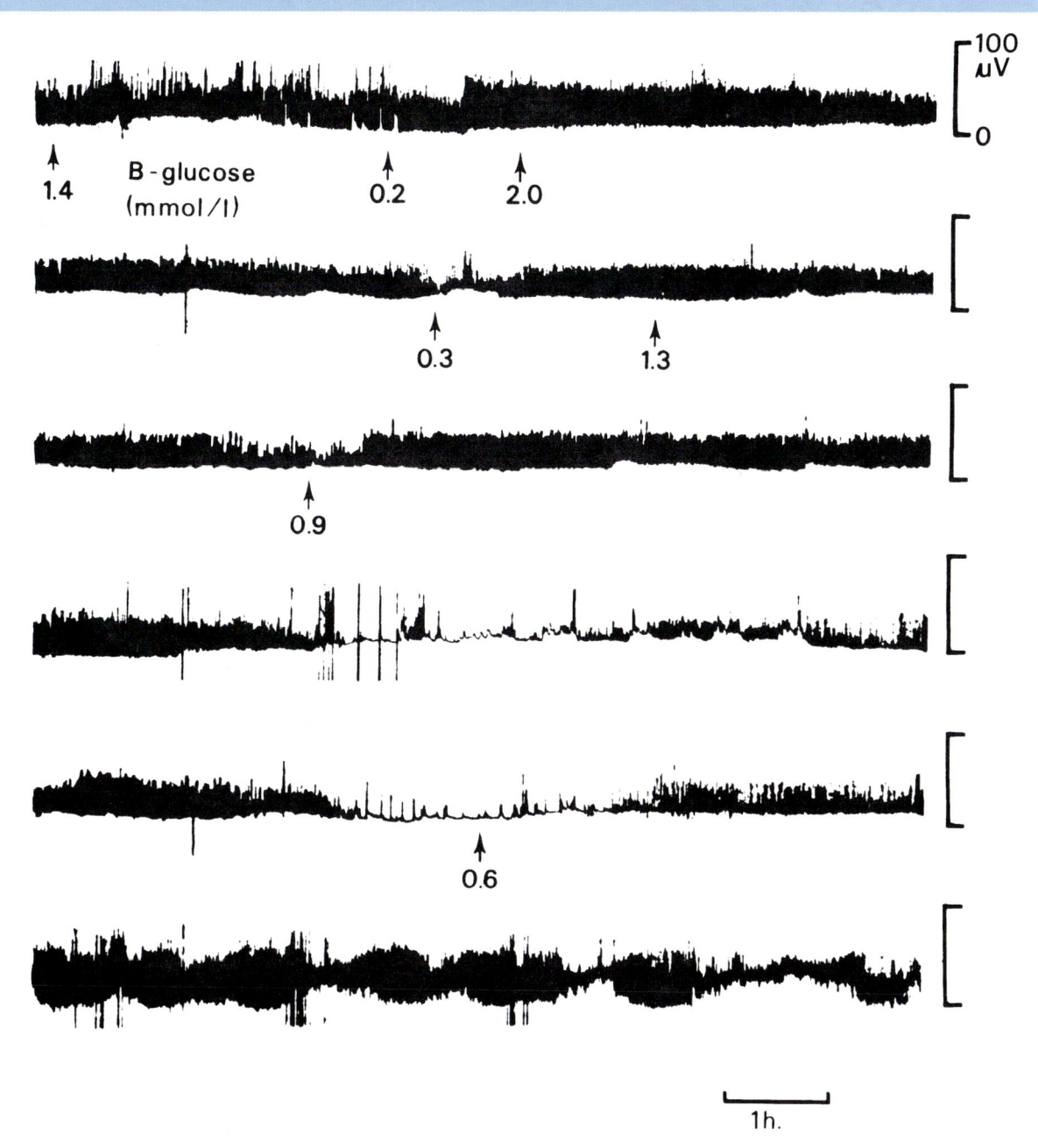

Figure 7.3 This was a female twin born at 38 weeks' gestation. Her birth weight was 2130 g and she was small for gestational age. On her 2nd day of life she developed septicemia and necrotizing enterocolitis. Her condition deteriorated and on the following day she needed mechanical ventilation and peritoneal dialysis. She was sedated and showed no specific clinical symptoms. She had aEEG as standard clinical monitoring.

The five upper aEEG traces represent 42 h of continuous monitoring starting on the infant's 4th day of life. The bottom tracing was recorded 1 week later. The aEEG background activity was initially discontinuous. On several occasions the background activity transiently deteriorated and became almost inactive during periods with hypoglycemia. During the first hours of the recording there were also a few suspected subclinical seizures before the blood glucose level of 0.2 mmol/l was recorded. One week later (bottom tracing), the electrocortical background had improved and was continuous with normal voltage and sleep–wake cycling. Reproduced from reference 50 with permission.

Periods with hypoglycemia may pass undetected in severely ill infants. The aEEG revealed the transient impact on brain function from the recurrent episodes of hypoglycemia

Hypoglycemia with seizures

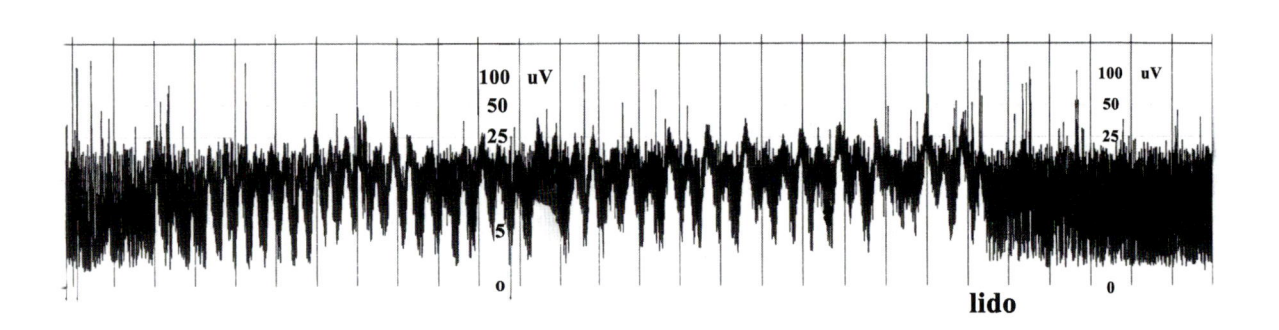

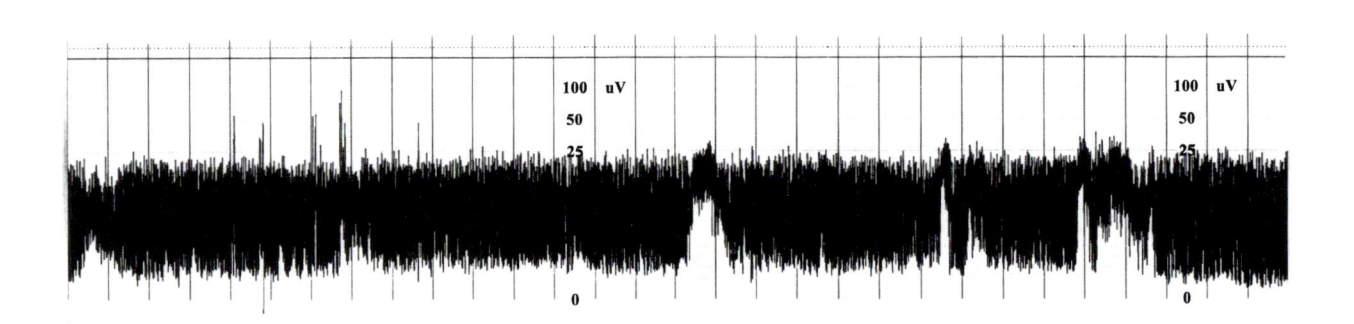

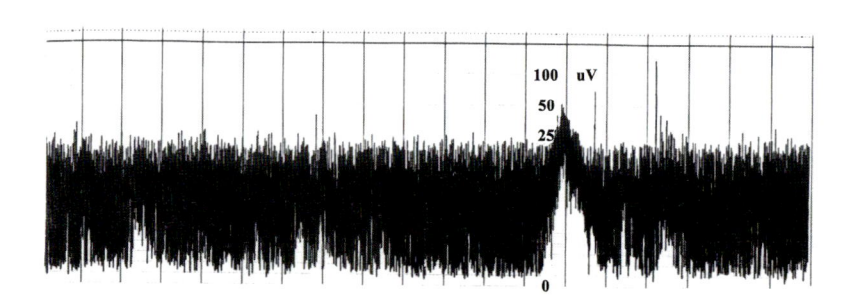

Figure 7.4 *opposite*   This male infant was born at 42 weeks' gestation following an uncomplicated pregnancy. He had a good start with Apgar scores of 8 and 10 at 1 and 5 min, respectively. At 24 h of age he was discharged home. Breastfeeding was slow and boiled water was given to guarantee his fluid intake. In the evening he was sweaty. He did not wake up during the night and the next morning he was found pale and cyanotic, and was difficult to wake. When he arrived at the hospital his blood glucose was zero, his breathing was shallow and his body temperature was 34°C. He was given intravenous glucose and a gradual rise in his blood glucose level was seen. From 3 h following admission he developed clinical seizures. Phenobarbitone, as well as phenytoin, were given, but failed to stop the clinical seizures. Twelve hours after admission he was admitted to the NICU with almost continuous clinical seizure activity. Clonazepam, which was given before transfer to the regional hospital, did not have any effect.

A cranial ultrasound performed on admission and a MRI at the end of the first week were unremarkable. His development was better than expected. His head circumference dropped from the 50th to the 10th centile but his motor development was within the normal range. At 6 years of age the MRI was repeated and once again was normal. His cognitive function was a little below the level for his age, and he was treated with valproate for epilepsy.

The aEEG was started on admission and showed a continuous seizure pattern ('saw-tooth'), with recurrent seizures every 2–3 min, concomitant with clinical seizures. The seizure pattern lasted for $3^1/_2$ hours, and was stopped temporarily by administration of lidocaine (lido; upper trace). The background activity after lidocaine was moderately discontinuous, but was not a burst-suppression pattern since the amplitude during the suppression periods (lower border of the trace) had an amplitude of 3–5 µV and some variability. After a few hours (middle and bottom traces), a few single subclinical seizures, lasting between a few minutes and up to 15 min, appeared in the recording. The aEEG backgound recovered over the following 24 h (not shown).

The normal MRI and cranial ultrasound scan in combination with the only moderately abnormal aEEG background were suggestive of a relatively good outcome in spite of the severe seizures. It is difficult to evaluate if the depressed aEEG background was due to the prior hypoglycemia or to the antiepileptic medications, or a combination of these factors

Continuous deterioration of aEEG background in an infant dying from a urea-cycle defect

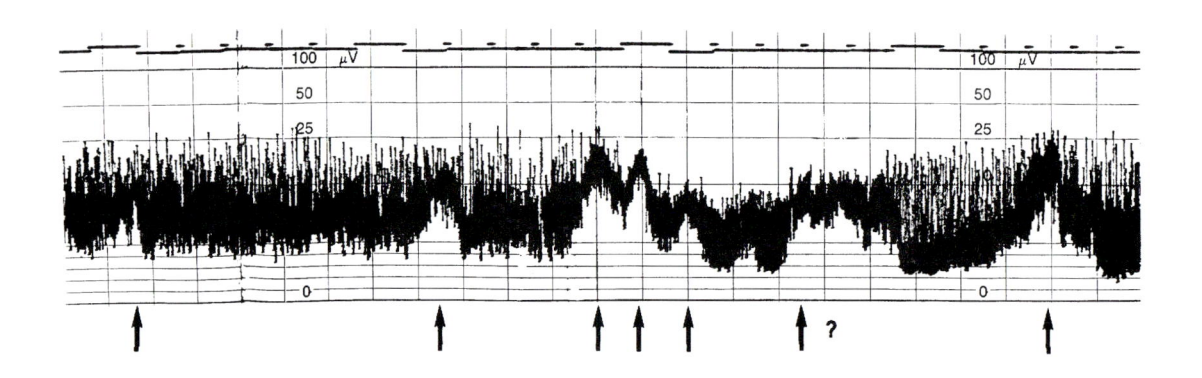

10 min

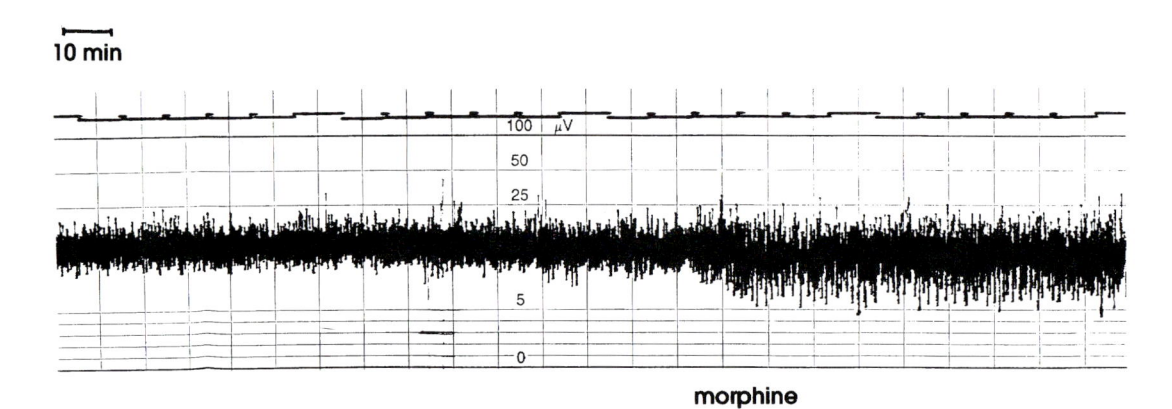

morphine

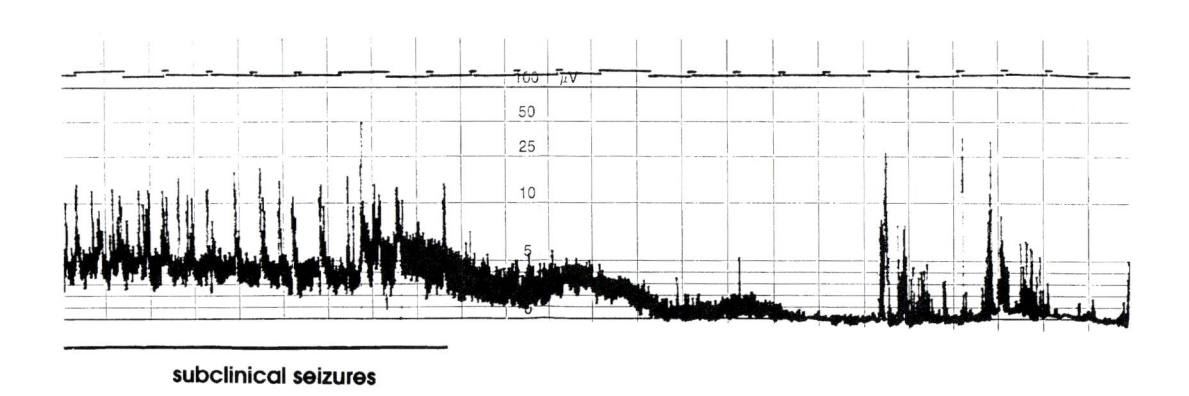

subclinical seizures

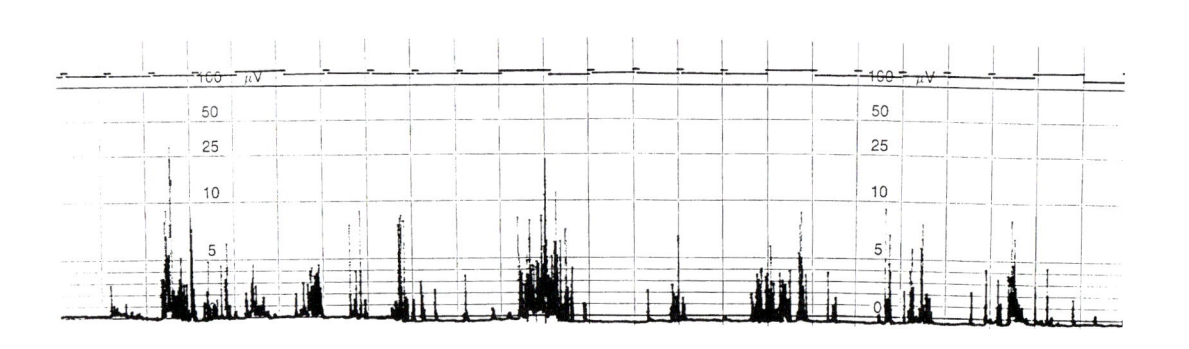

Figure 7.5 *opposite*   This was a full-term female infant, born by normal vaginal delivery following an uncomplicated pregnancy. On her 3rd day of life she was admitted to the NICU with clonic seizures. Clinical investigations showed high blood ammonium levels, and a urea-cycle defect was suspected. Peritoneal dialysis was initiated and she was treated with arginine. Her condition did not improve in spite of the treatment and she died at the age of 13 days.

The aEEG tracing started when she was admitted to the NICU at the age of 3 days (top trace). The aEEG background was slightly periodic but became more discontinuous at the end of this trace. The arrows indicate clinical seizures corresponding to seizure activity in the aEEG. At the question mark, clinical seizures had ceased but the aEEG showed suspected seizure activity for 15–20 min.

The second trace was recorded 4 days later, on day 7. The infant was on mechanical ventilation and had not improved clinically, even though the ammonium levels were lower. The aEEG background was continuous but showed very little variability. The background amplitude decreased moderately after morphine administration.

At the third trace she was 11 days old and no clinical improvement was noted. At the start, the aEEG showed a period with subclinical seizure activity that ceased spontaneously. After the cessation of seizure activity, the electrocortical background deteriorated further and became inactive.

The aEEG did not recover and was still inactive at 13 days (fourth trace); at that time it only showed interference during caregiving. The infant died later the same day.

This recording shows that it is possible to follow closely, and for a long duration, the cerebral activity with aEEG. Even though evaluation of brain death is difficult in newborn infants, the aEEG is suggestive of the timing in this infant (third trace)

Effect of mixed acidosis in a stable newborn piglet

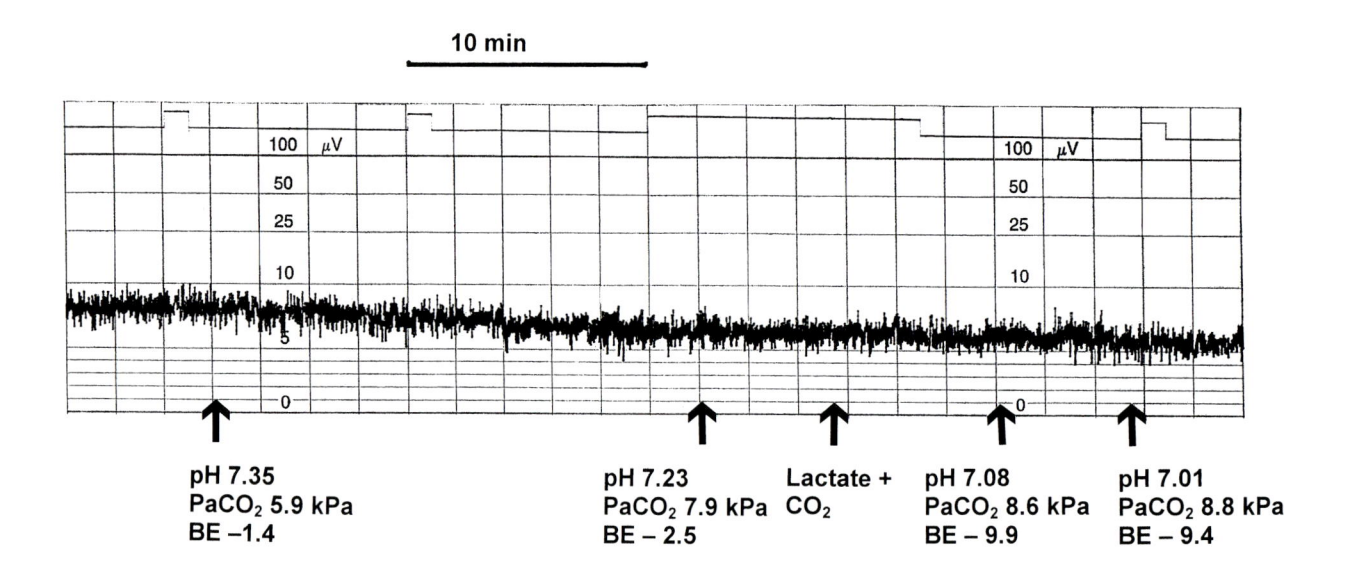

Figure 7.6   The effect on the neonatal EEG from acidosis has not been extensively studied. A study by Eaton and colleagues, using another type of EEG monitoring, indicated that reversible background changes due to acidosis could be diagnosed with EEG monitoring[146]. The effect on the aEEG from mixed acidosis was studied in newborn piglets[147]. The piglets were anesthetized with halothane and fentanyl. They received an infusion with lactic acid and, simultaneously, carbon dioxide was added to the inspired gas mixture, resulting in a mixed acidosis. This piglet was accidentally under-ventilated before the lactic acid and carbon dioxide were given, and the pH decreased from 7.35 to 7.23 while the $PaCO_2$ rose from 5.9 kPa to 7.9 kPa. After adding lactic acid and carbon dioxide the pH fell to 7.01 and the $PaCO_2$ rose to 8.8 kPa.

The aEEG was recorded at a slow speed (30 cm/h). The initial tracing is a continuous background pattern with relatively low amplitude. The aEEG amplitude decreased in parallel with the decreasing pH and increasing $PaCO_2$. The simultaneously recorded raw EEG (not shown) showed a decrease in fast frequencies. Mixed acidosis does seem to have some influence on aEEG background in an experimental setting. However, in a clinical situation the impact from acidosis on the aEEG is more uncertain

Non-ketotic hyperglycinemia

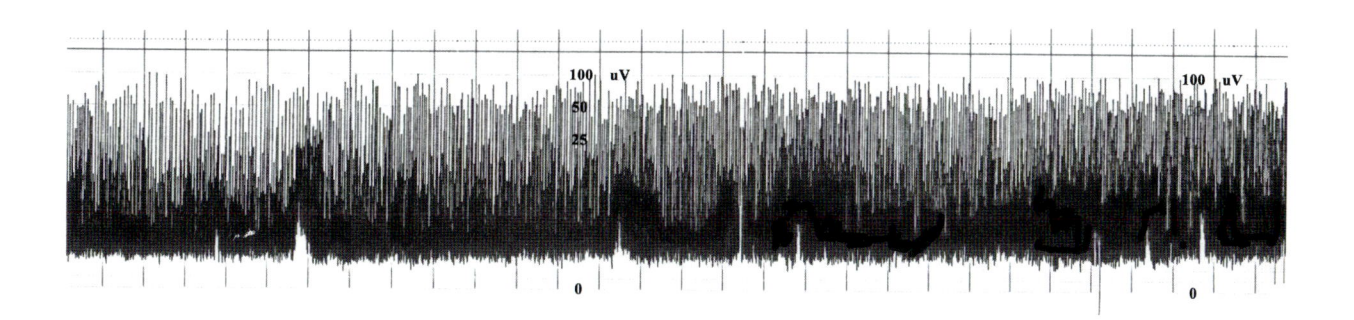

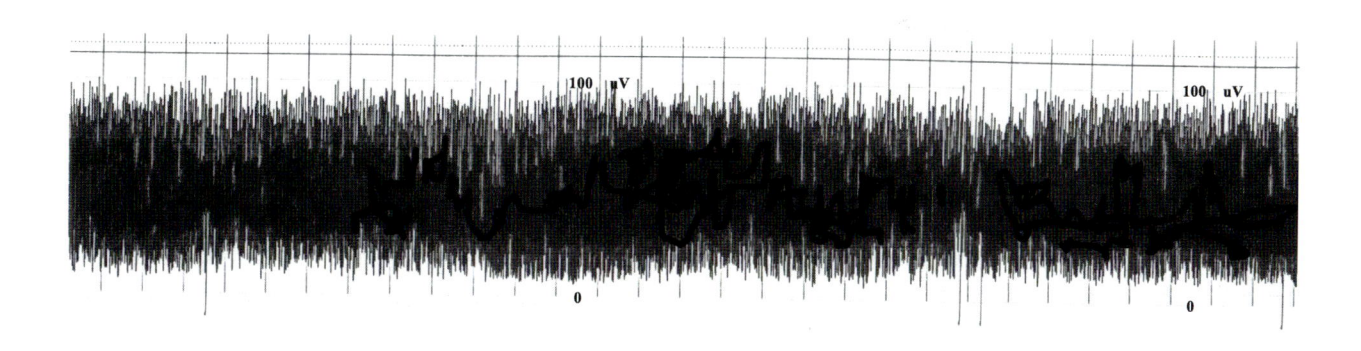

Figure 7.7 This female infant was born as the fourth child, the previous three children all being healthy. The pregnancy was uneventful and she was delivered at home at 39 weeks' gestation, weighing 3100 g. She did not feed very well and developed vomiting and oliguria. On the 4th day, she was hypothermic and the mother could not wake her. She was admitted to the local hospital and suspected of having septicemia. At the hospital she developed seizures and received phenobarbitone. As she required mechanical ventilation she was transferred to the NICU. On admission she was comatose with occasional clinical seizures. The cranial ultrasound examination showed dysgenesis of the corpus callosum. A metabolic work-up was carried out and the diagnosis of non-ketotic hyperglycinemia was made.

The aEEG was started and showed a burst-suppression pattern. Burst suppression is a typical feature of non-ketotic hyperglycinemia[137,138], but is also a non-specific marker of brain dysfunction. The aEEG and EEG cannot be used for diagnosing this metabolic disease. Initially, in the upper tracing there were a few transient increases in the background activity, with duration of 1–4 min. These background changes are suspected as being epileptic seizure activity. On the lower trace, a slight improvement of the background has occurred with some variability of the minimum amplitude and without suspected seizure activity

Mitochondrial disorder

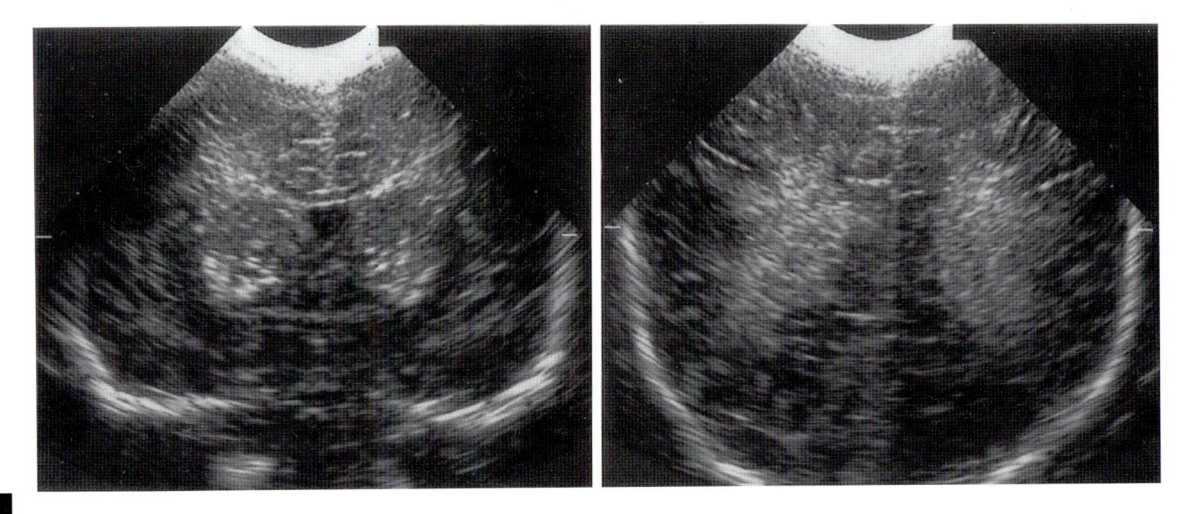

a

Figure 7.8 *above and opposite* This male infant was born at 42 weeks' gestation. He was the second affected child of related parents. The first child also died in the neonatal period with the diagnosis of a respiratory chain defect (complex I deficiency). This boy developed apneic spells within 1 h of delivery and was intubated. His chest X-ray showed a large heart, and cardiac ultrasound examination showed signs of severe cardiomyopathy. Serum lactate levels varied between 10 and 20 mmol/l. He required increasing inotropic support, but died due to cardiac failure on the 2nd day of life.

(a) The cranial ultrasound scan shows areas of calcification in the basal ganglia. Similar changes had also been present in the sibling. Increased echogenicity was also seen in the periventricular white matter.

(b) The aEEG recording was started at 3 h of age and showed a DNV pattern with variability suggestive of sleep–wake cycling. Two clinical seizures (asterisks), and one period with lower oxygen saturation (sa), were present in the upper part of the recording but no clear seizure activity could be identified on the aEEG. A marked depression of the background activity was seen following administration of midazolam (middle trace). The continuous background became discontinuous with burst suppression. A suspected seizure pattern emerges after the midazolam. The suspected seizure pattern is quite subtle, and is represented by small but regular increases in the minimum amplitude coinciding with transient decreases in burst density. When this pattern had been present for a little more than 1 h it was interrupted after a clinical seizure (asterisk). A similar pattern can be seen at the beginning of the bottom trace. A few single transient increases in the minimum amplitude occur later and are also suspected as being seizure activity although they could also represent reaction to care procedures

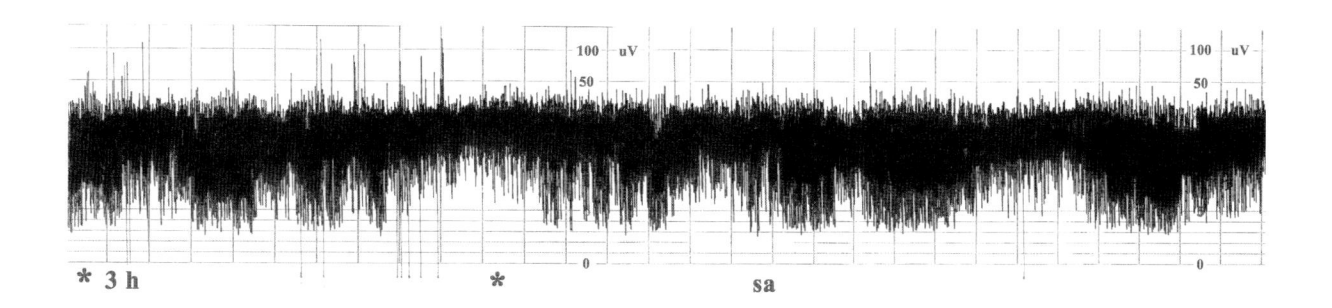

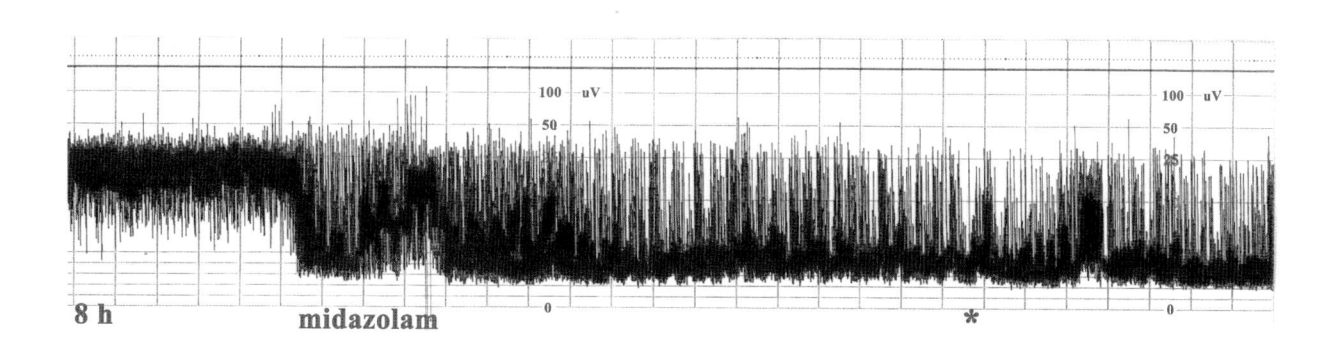

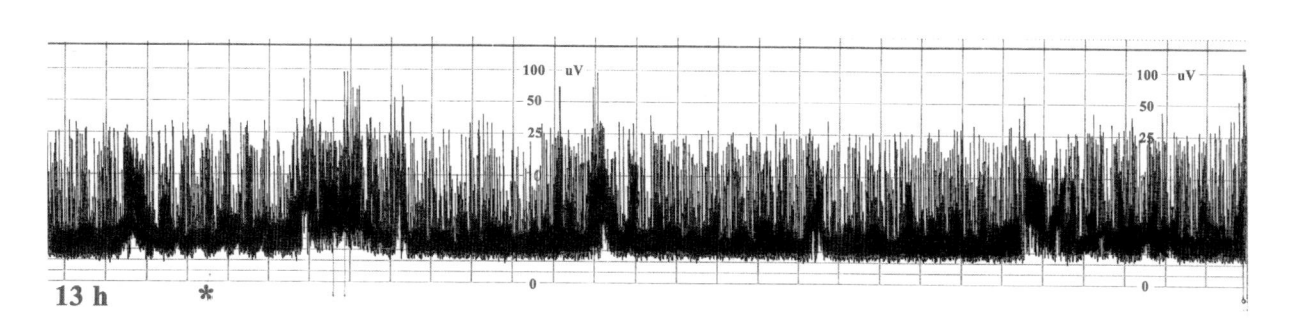

b

Pyridoxine-responsive seizures

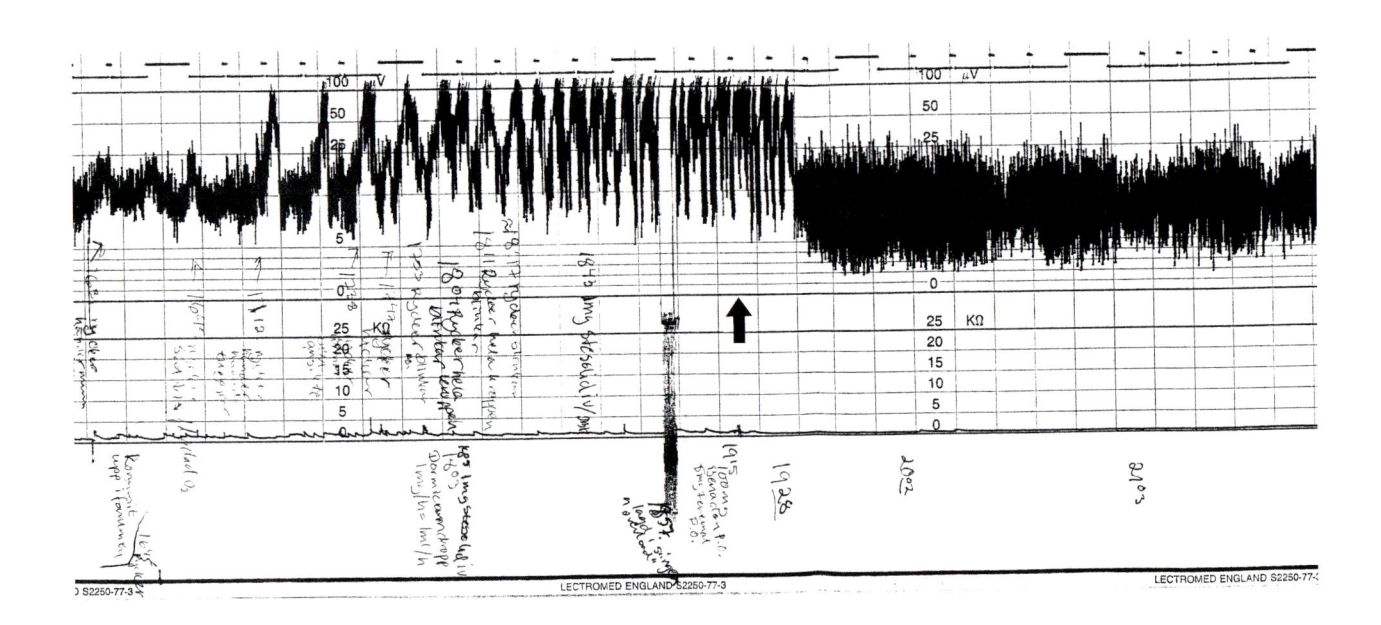

Figure 7.9   This full-term male infant was born after a normal pregnancy with Apgar scores of 9, 9 and 10, an umbilical artery pH of 7.21 and meconium-stained amniotic fluid. He was admitted to the neonatal unit because he was irritable and had moderate metabolic acidosis. Myoclonic seizures started at 12 h and continued for several days in spite of treatment with diazepam, phenobarbitone, lidocaine and phenytoin. A CT scan and a metabolic work-up were normal. Two standard EEGs were performed and showed burst suppression and normal activity. He recovered after 12 days but the seizures recurred when he developed suspected septicemia some days later. Again, antiepileptic treatment with diazepam, phenobarbitone, lidocaine and phenytoin did not stop the seizures. The pyridoxine was given with immediate effect on the seizure activity (see below). At the age of 8 years he had developed moderate mental retardation. He has continued with pyridoxine, and a decision to withdraw the pyridoxine was changed when very subtle episodes of arrested activity occurred with a corresponding left-sided rhythmic theta activity on the EEG. He has a younger sibling with pyridoxine-respondent neonatal seizures.

The aEEG was recorded when the seizures recurred at 15 days. The recurrent clinical and concomitant electrographic seizures can be seen as a 'saw-tooth' pattern during the first 4 h of the tracing. The seizures were totally abolished 15 min after 100 mg pyridoxine was given orally (at the arrow) through the nasogastric feeding tube (there was no intravenous pyridoxine available). After the administration of the pyridoxine the aEEG showed continuous background activity with a slightly periodic pattern (low minimum amplitude but normal maximum voltage) and cyclical fluctuations suggestive of sleep–wake cycling. Reproduced from reference 142 with permission

Pyridoxine-dependent seizures in a preterm infant

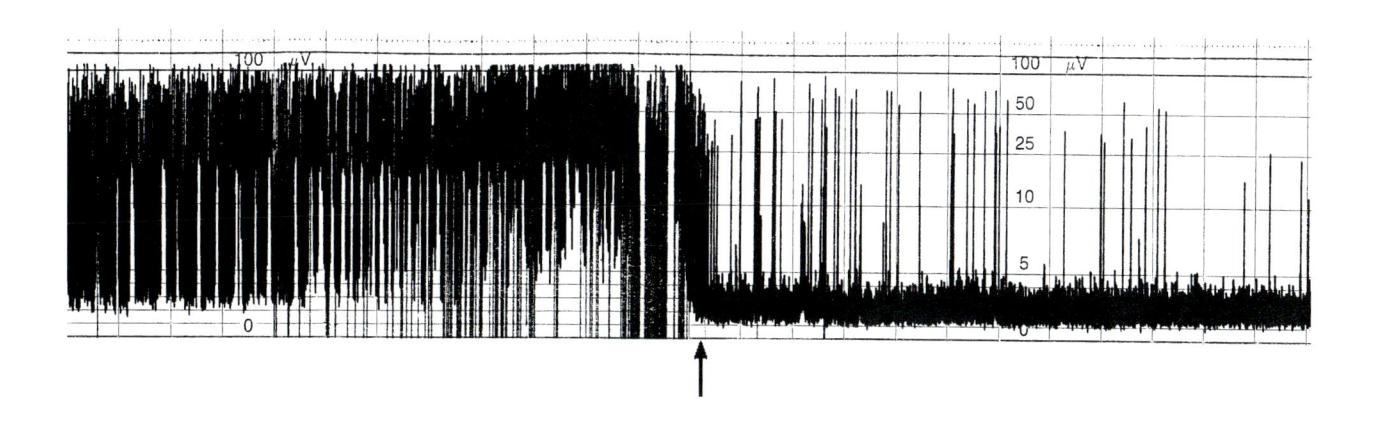

Figure 7.10 This female infant was born at 34 weeks' gestation with Apgar scores 6, 8 and 9 at 1, 5 and 10 min, respectively, and a birth weight of 2240 g. A routine ultrasound examination at 32 weeks' gestation showed bowel dilatation, otherwise the pregnancy was normal. Soon after birth the infant became restless and irritable. Abdominal ultrasound scans and X-rays were normal. She had a metabolic acidosis with a pH of 7.08, base excess of –21 mmol/l, and plasma lactate level of 20 mmol/l. At 12 h she needed sedation (with midazolam and morphine) and mechanical ventilation due to the irritability. On the 3rd day of life she developed multifocal myoclonic seizures. She received intravenous diazepam and lidocaine with no effect, and was then given 100 mg pyridoxine intravenously. The seizures stopped within 2 min, and she became profoundly hypotonic. A standard EEG on the following day was discontinuous with bilateral epileptiform activity, but the EEG normalized within 3 days. She had no more seizures and was extubated after 5 days. A trial of pyridoxine withdrawal was carried out when she was aged 2.5 years, and resulted in recurrent seizures and continuing pyridoxine medication. Her development is slightly delayed.

The aEEG showed high-amplitude recurrent, almost continuous, electrographic seizure activity concomitant with the clinical seizures. After pyridoxine administration (at arrow) the aEEG changed dramatically, the electrographic seizure activity ceased almost immediately and the background amplitude became extremely low in voltage. The aEEG background recovered slowly during the following 8–10 h. Reproduced from reference 142 with permission

Bacterial encephalitis

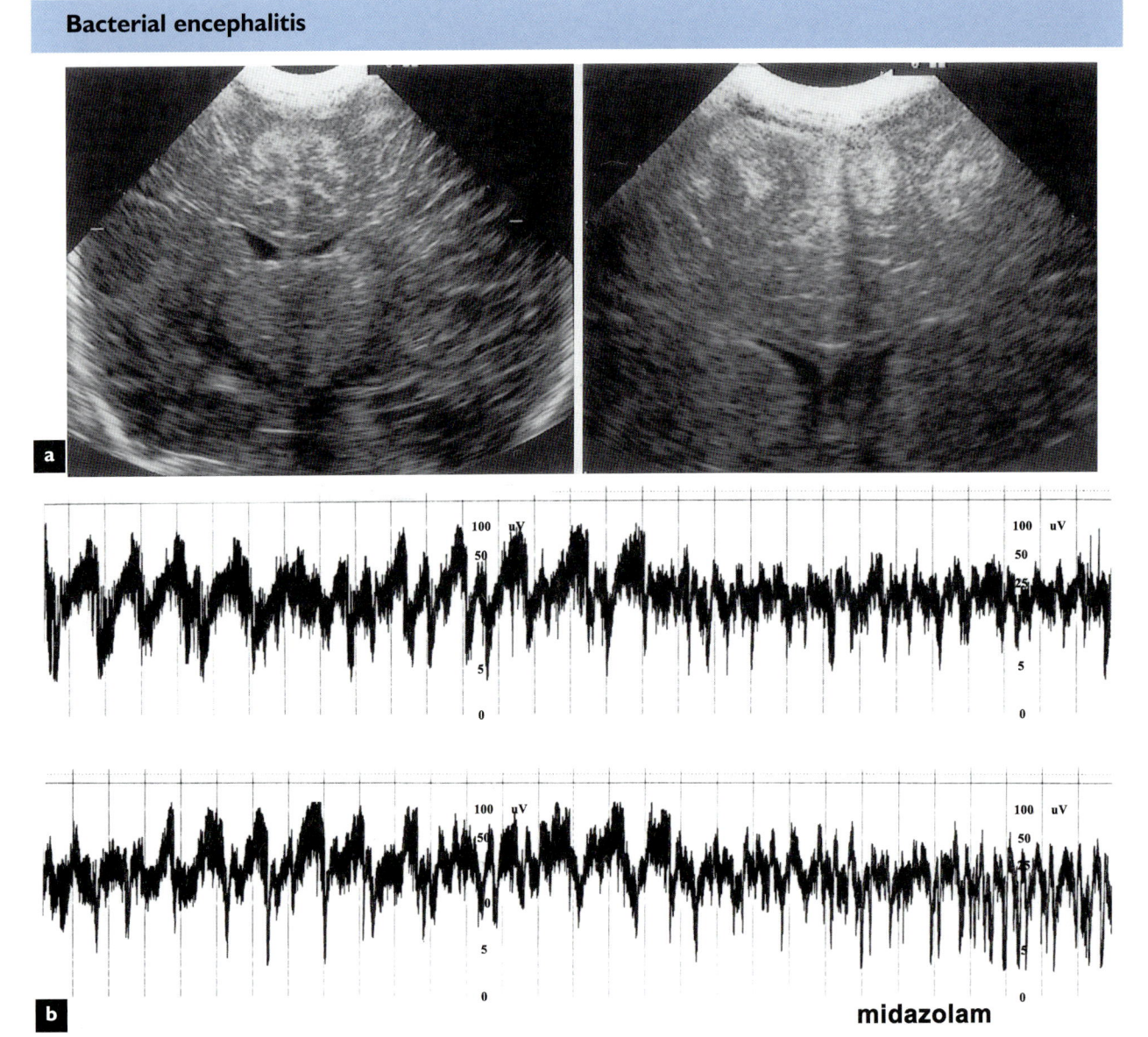

Figure 7.11 *above and opposite* This male infant was born at term and did not have any perinatal problems. He was admitted when he was 6 weeks old with fever and focal seizures. He was given a loading dose of phenobarbitone which stopped the clinical seizures. Antibiotics were started once a blood culture and lumbar puncture were carried out. He was intubated because of inadequate ventilation and was then transferred to the pediatric intensive care unit. *Pneumococci* were cultured from the blood and cerebrospinal fluid. His fontanelle was tense and his eyes deviated to the left. He remained unresponsive. Intensive care treatment was withdrawn in view of the poor prognosis. Permission for a postmortem examination was not obtained.

(a) Cranial ultrasound examination using a 7.5- and a 10-MHz transducer showed severe diffuse echogenicity, especially marked in the cortex and subcortical white matter and the thalami.

(b) The long aEEG recording showed several periods with repetitive seizure activity corresponding with subclinical status epilepticus. The frequency and duration of individual seizures varied during the recording. Midazolam did not have any effect on the seizure pattern. However, lidocaine temporarily stopped the status epilepticus and a burst-suppression background pattern was seen for 6–8 h before the electrographic seizures recurred with increasing intensity (traces 4–8). Two standard EEGs were recorded at times when the seizure activity was controlled and showed burst suppression but no ongoing seizure activity.

This example shows the advantages of, and the additional information that is obtained with, a long-term continuous recording, even if it is simplified as in the aEEG

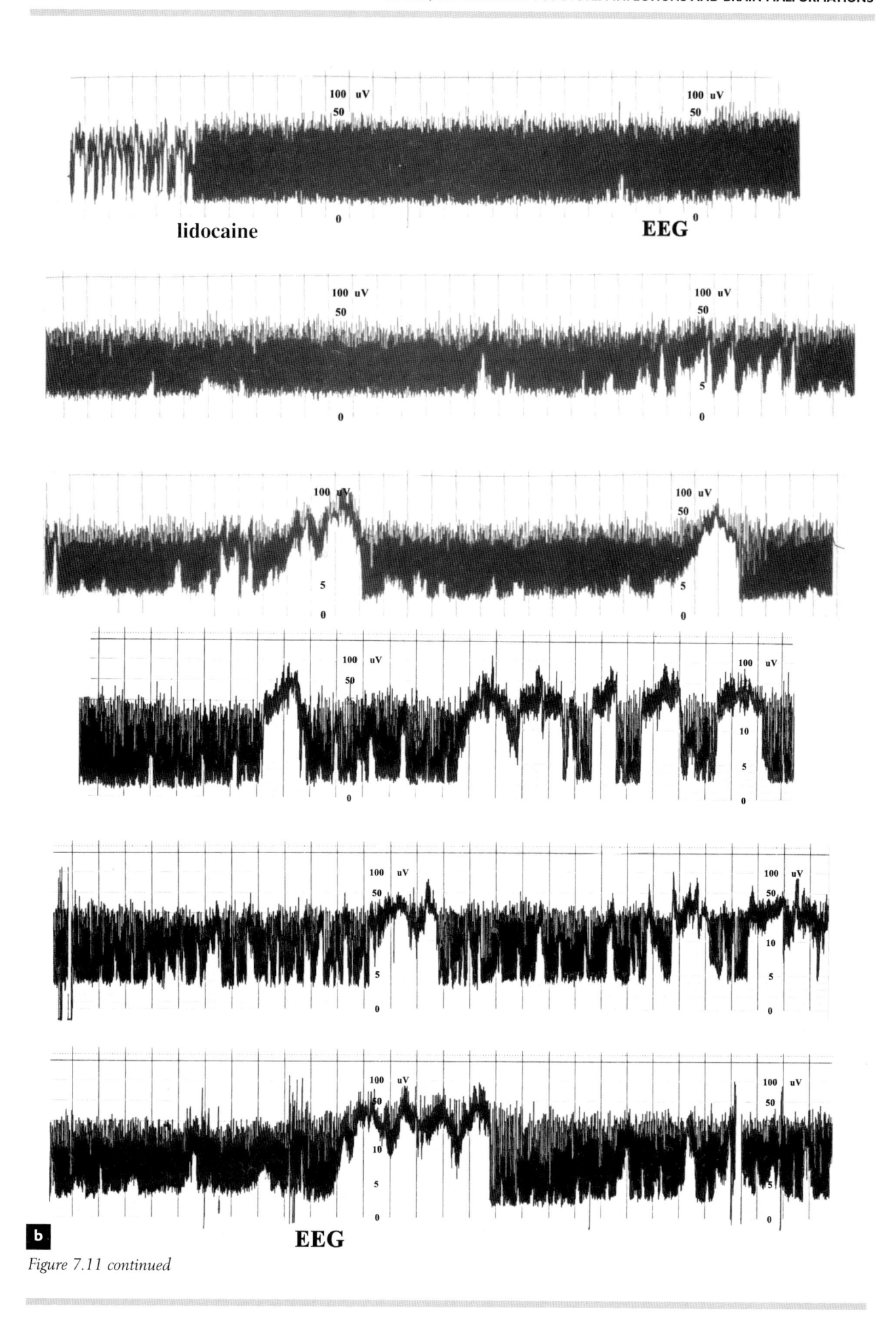

Figure 7.11 continued

Group B streptococcus meningitis

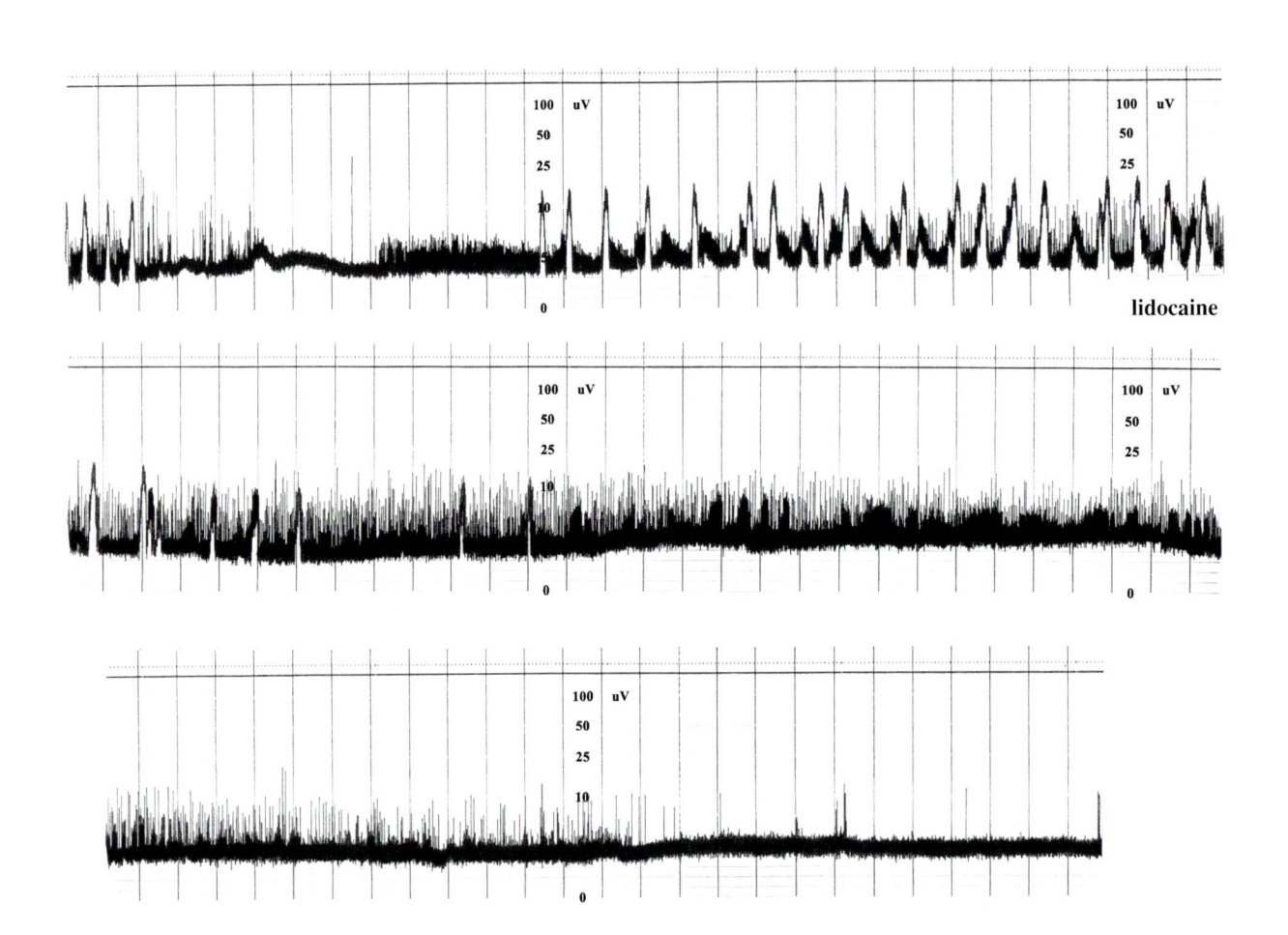

Figure 7.12 This male infant was born following a home delivery at 36 weeks' gestation. When he was $2^1/_2$ weeks old, he suddenly became ill with poor feeding and fever. He was initially admitted to a local hospital where he was found to have a bulging fontanelle, tachycardia (200–220/min) and developed apneas. He was intubated and a lumbar puncture was performed. He received antibiotics and was transferred to the NICU. He was severely hypotensive on arrival and in spite of increasing inotropic support (dopamine, dobutamine and hydrocortisone) died the next day following further cardiovascular deterioration. The cerebrospinal fluid cultures were positive for group B streptococci.

The initial aEEG showed recurrent low-amplitude epileptic seizure activity on an inactive background. At the beginning of the recording three seizures can be seen and then the seizure pattern ceased spontaneously and recurred $1^1/_2$ h later. Following administration of lidocaine, a few more seizures were present and the background activity remained extremely low in amplitude. On the middle trace, a low-amplitude burst-suppression pattern with decreasing amplitude is present and on the bottom trace the background becomes inactive. The depressed electrocortical background was predictive of the poor outcome in this infant, as shown also in other newborn infants with bacterial meningitis[148]

Systemic herpes infection with encephalitis

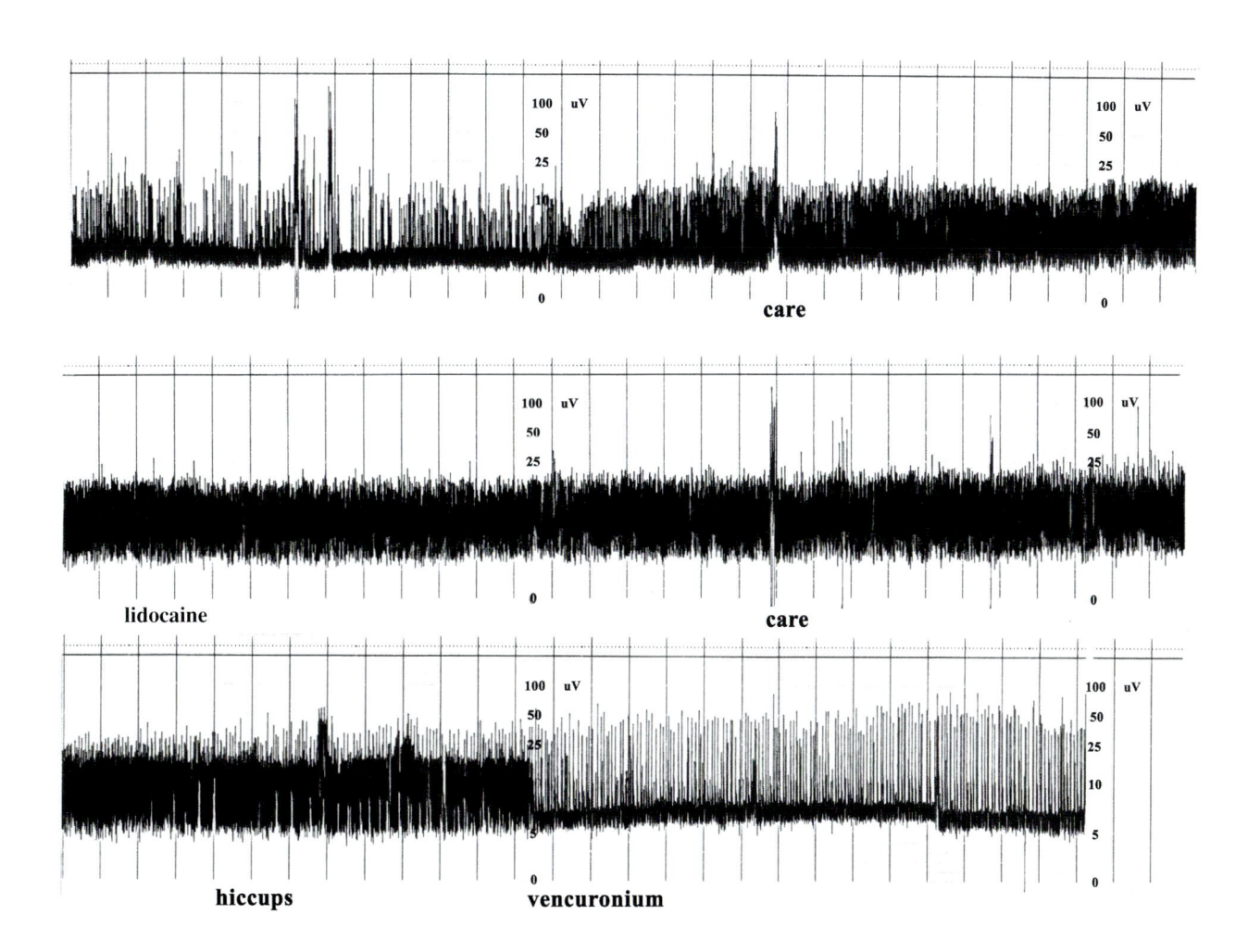

Figure 7.13 This male infant was born at 40 weeks' gestation, following an uncomplicated delivery. His birth weight was 3340 g and he had good Apgar scores. On day 6 he developed a fever (38.6°C) and was admitted to hospital. Following blood culture and a lumbar culture he was started on antibiotics. His clinical condition deteriorated and the next day he needed mechanical ventilation. He was noted to ooze from puncture sites and had severely prolonged clotting times. He also developed clinical seizures and received phenobarbitone. At this stage herpes infection was suspected although there was no parental history to support this, but cultures from the nose and throat grew herpes simplex type I. He was transferred to the NICU but in spite of extensive support he deteriorated and died.

The aEEG showed a low-voltage burst-suppression pattern with short transient increases in the minimum and maximum amplitudes during care procedures, which could be due to arousals or movement artefacts. There appears to be some improvement of the background activity with increased burst density and a slight rise in the minimum amplitudes. He received lidocaine (middle trace) for suspected seizures, although no clear seizure activity can be detected in the aEEG. He developed increasingly irregular respiration and hiccups, associated with transient rises in the aEEG background (lower tracing). As there was suspicion that the hiccups affected the background pattern, vencuronium (a muscle relaxant) was given. It is clear that this was the case, since a sparse burst-suppression pattern reappeared after the vencuronium

Incontinentia pigmenti

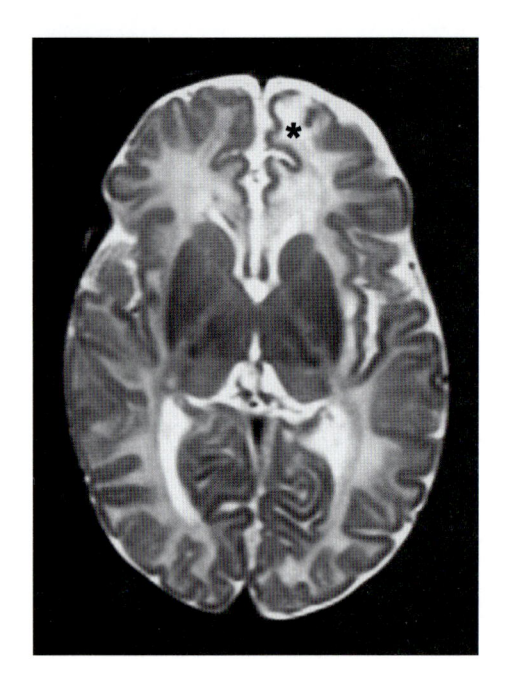
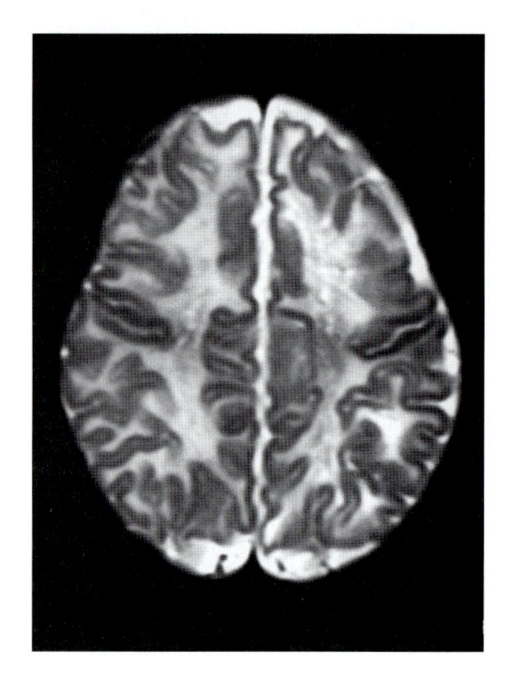

a

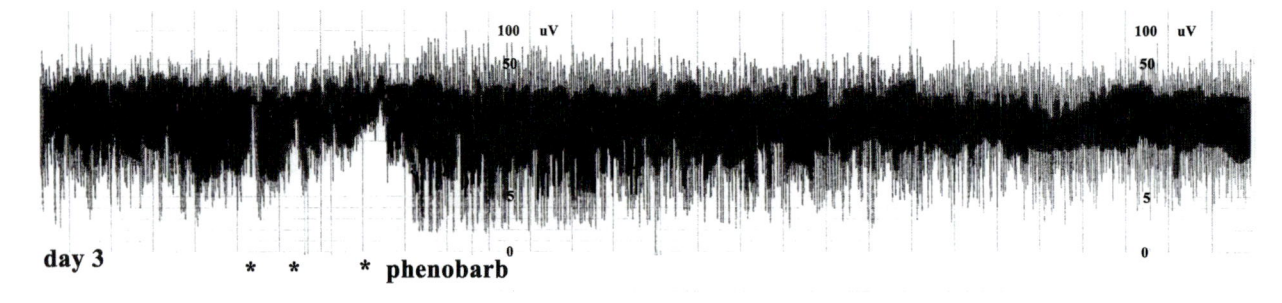

day 3   *   *   * phenobarb

b

Figure 7.14   This female infant was born at 39 weeks' gestation following a normal delivery. No problems were noted initially, but on day 3 she was admitted to hospital with clinical seizures.

Cranial ultrasound examination on admission showed subcortical echogenicity, which was especially marked on the left side. By day 10, small cystic lesions were identified in this left-sided echogenic area.

(a) MRI confirmed an area of high-signal intensity on T_2-weighted inversion recovery sequence in the left frontal lobe, extending into the deep subcortical white matter (asterisk) and more diffuse changes throughout the centrum semiovale, compatible with leukomalacia. By 2 weeks of age, typical linear skin lesions were noted, and the ophthalmologist diagnosed eye abnormalities typical for incontinentia pigmenti. The perinatal history, which was uneventful, in combination with the skin and eye abnormalities led to the diagnosis. Reproduced from reference 149 with permission.

(b) The aEEG background activity was mainly continuous. However, since the minimum amplitude was low (< 5 μV) on several occasions, this means that the background activity was slightly discontinuous and contained short periods with low voltage activity, a DNV pattern. The infant had three clinical seizures (asterisks), with corresponding changes in the aEEG, seen as transient lifts of the baseline. Phenobarbitone was effective in treating the seizures. The antiepileptic medication also affected the background activity which became more discontinuous, although at the end of the tracing the background pattern has recovered. There are no specific aEEG changes in incontinentia pigmenti

Tuberous sclerosis

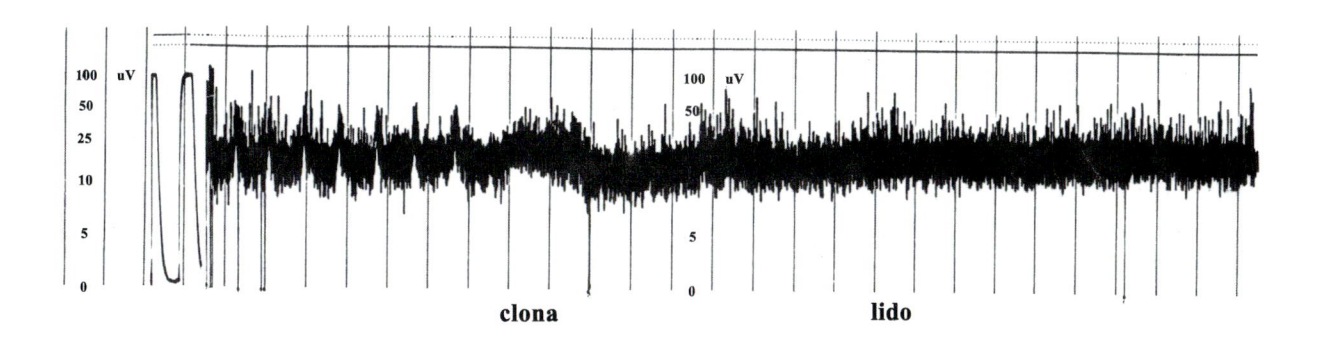

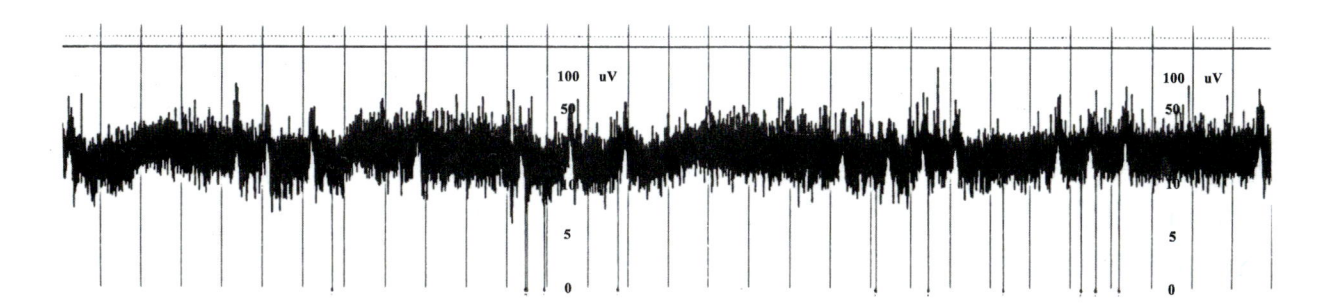

Figure 7.15 This male infant was born at 39 weeks' gestation by emergency Cesarean section following two failed ventouse extractions. His Apgar scores were 3, 7 and 7 at 1, 5 and 10 min, respectively, and his birth weight was 3640 g. He was admitted to the special care baby unit and was given phenobarbitone following the onset of clinical generalized seizures occurring on day 1. The seizures were difficult to control and he also received clonazepam. He was initially discharged at 3 weeks of age, but 4 days later his mother could not wake him and he was readmitted. Clinical seizures were still present and phenytoin was added to the medication. He developed a suspected hemorrhage in the basal ganglia on the right and was transferred to the NICU at the age of 4 weeks. On admission he had frequent clonic seizures. A cranial ultrasound examination showed an area of increased echogenicity of different intensity in the right striatum and some subcortical echogenic areas. A cardiac ultrasound revealed five large rhabdomyomas. A CT scan confirmed the suspected tuberous sclerosis with subcortical tubers and a hamartoma in the basal ganglia.

The aEEG background activity was continuous with normal voltage and showed some variability but no clear sleep–wake cycling. At the beginning of the recording there are seven clinical seizures with corresponding seizure activity in the aEEG. The seizures were temporarily interrupted by administration of clonazepam and lidocaine but recurred some hours later. The infant was then referred to the neuropediatric ward

Hemimegalencephaly

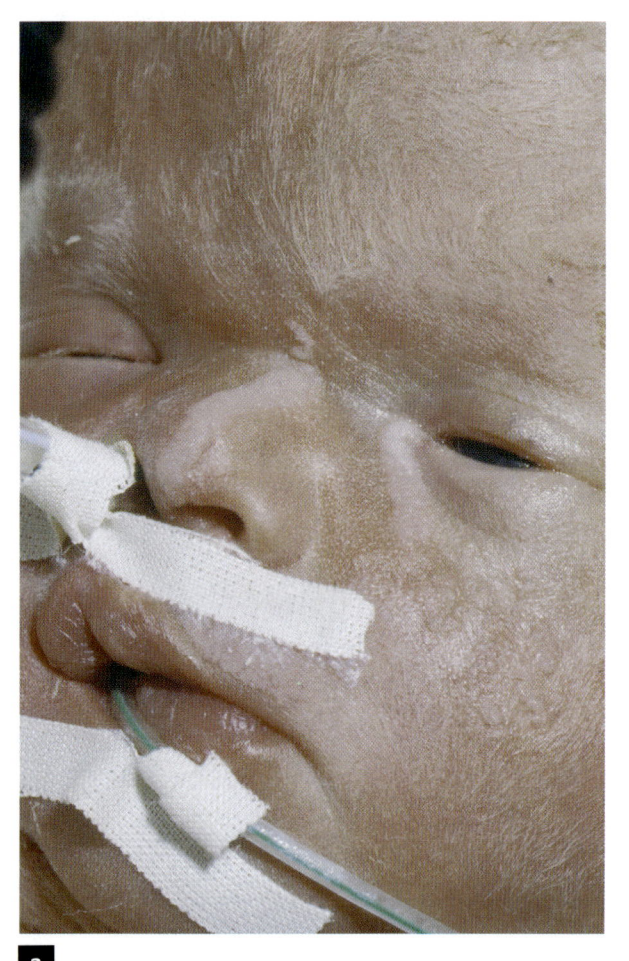

Figure 7.16 This male infant was born at 32 weeks' gestation. Antenatal ultrasonography had shown a dilated left lateral ventricle. His Apgar scores were 4 at 1 min and 5 at 5 min. He was intubated and transferred to the NICU. His birth weight was 2620 g (97th centile) and his head circumference was 38 cm (97th centile).

(a) He had an asymmetrical skull and a linear nevus sebaceus over the nose and under the left eye. Reproduced from reference 145 with permission.

(b) A cranial ultrasound examination (coronal and parasagittal view) confirmed the dilatation of the left lateral ventricle which was irregular in shape. Areas of increased echogenicity were present surrounding the ventricle, suggestive of calcification. This was subsequently confirmed by a CT scan. The infant received the diagnosis of Jadassohn syndrome, a syndrome that includes partial seizures or infantile spasms, mental retardation, hemimacrocrania and ocular abnormalitites. Intensive care was withdrawn.

(c) Permission for a postmortem examination was given and hemimegalencephaly was confirmed. A coronal slice of the brain shows a very large polygonal left lateral ventricle, with several periventricular cysts and areas of calcification. There is severe thickening of the cortex

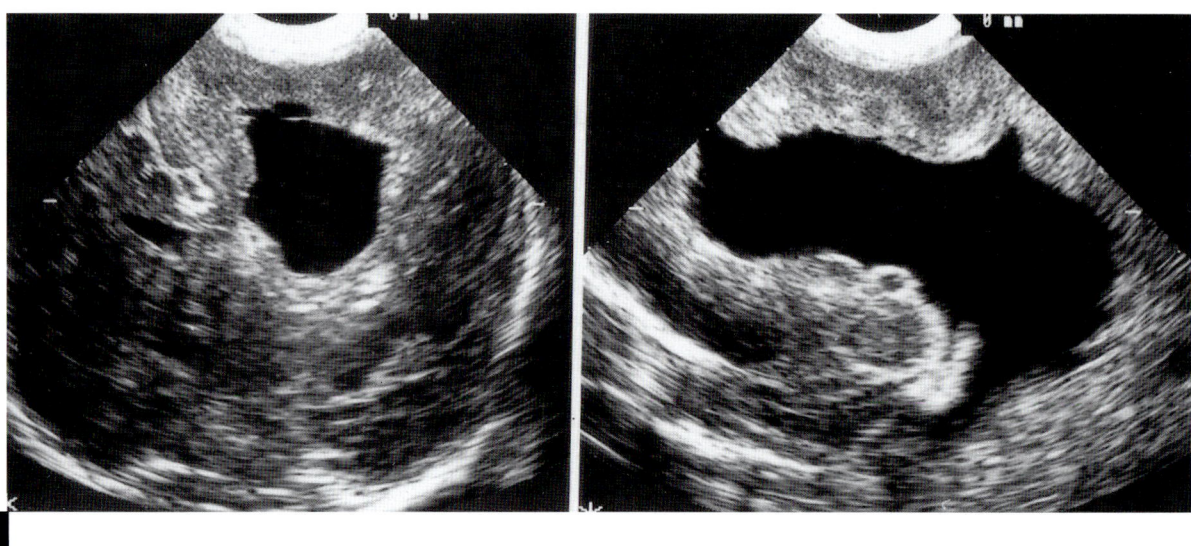

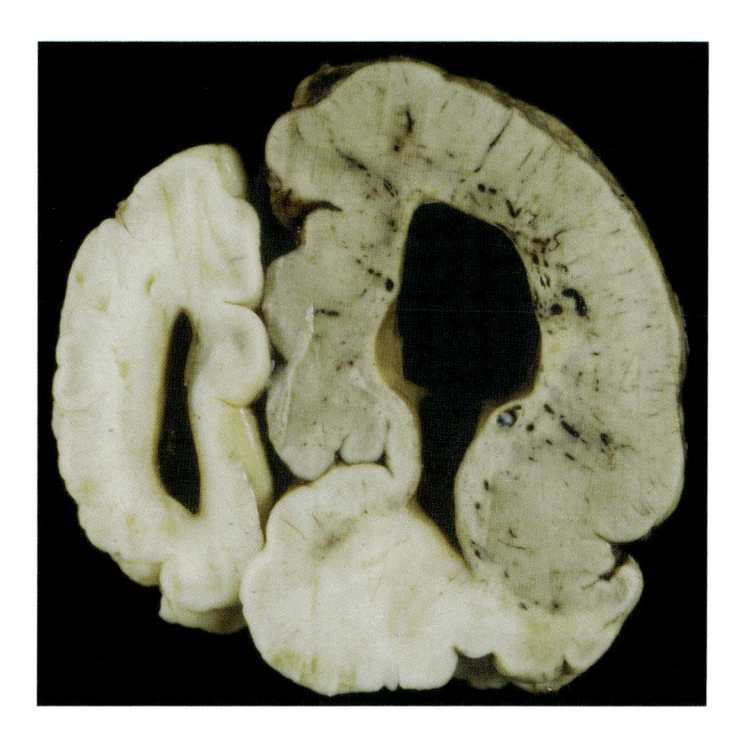

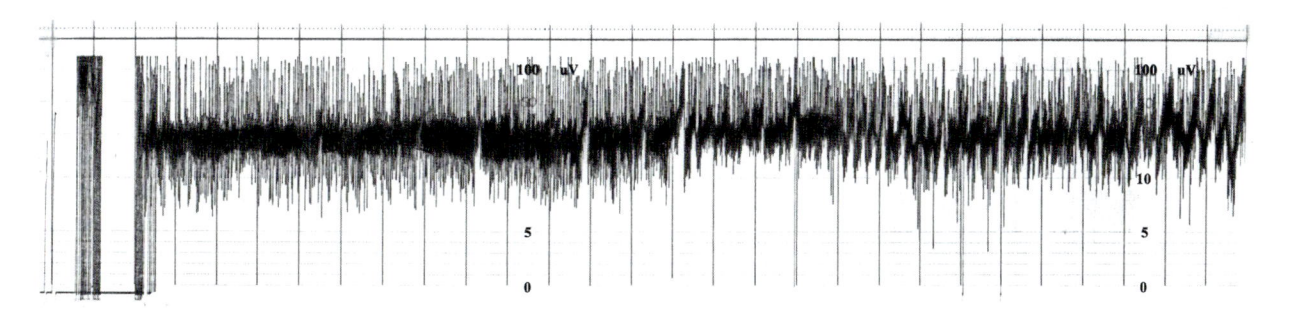

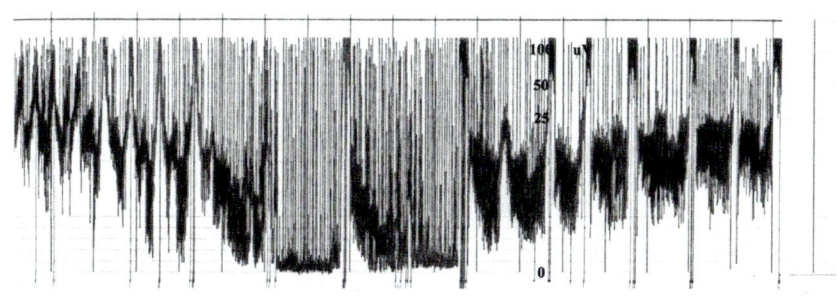

clonazepam

Figure 7.16 continued   (d) The aEEG was started soon after birth. However, it was impossible to receive a conventional biparietal recording (P3–P4) due to continuous overload (see the very short initial recording that was interrupted). One reason why it was impossible to record from the standard leads could be that epileptic seizure acitivty in Jadassohn syndrome may be of very high amplitude. When a P3–F3 recording (frontal–parietal leads on the left side) was carried out an abnormal high-voltage backgound pattern was first present with increasing intensity of repetitive electrical seizures ('saw-tooth' pattern). Clonazepam briefly interrupted the seizure pattern

Suspected hereditary hemorrhagic telangiectasia (Osler–Weber–Rendu syndrome)

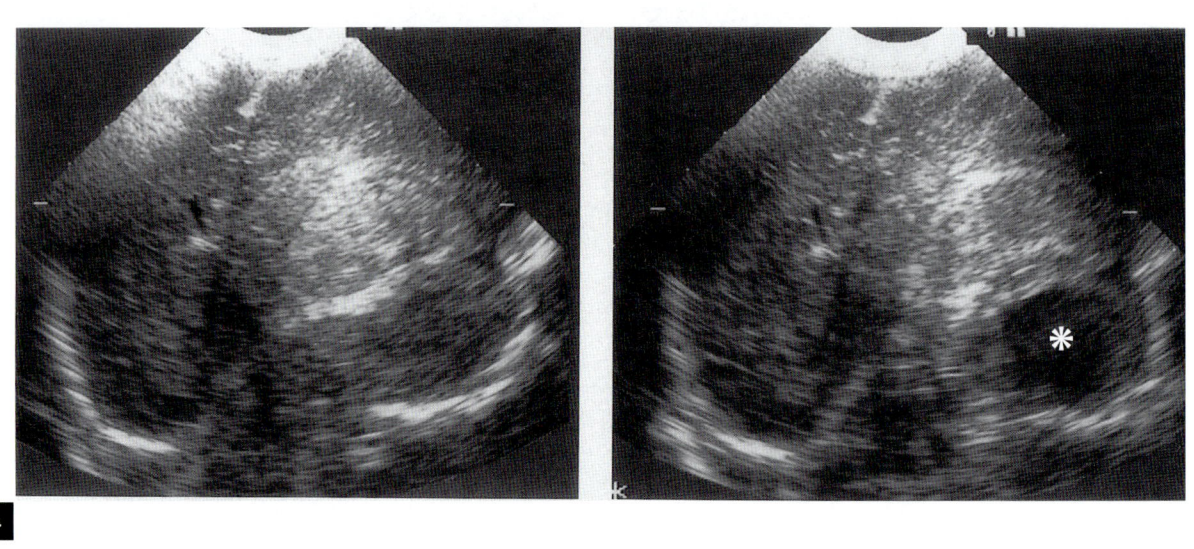

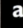

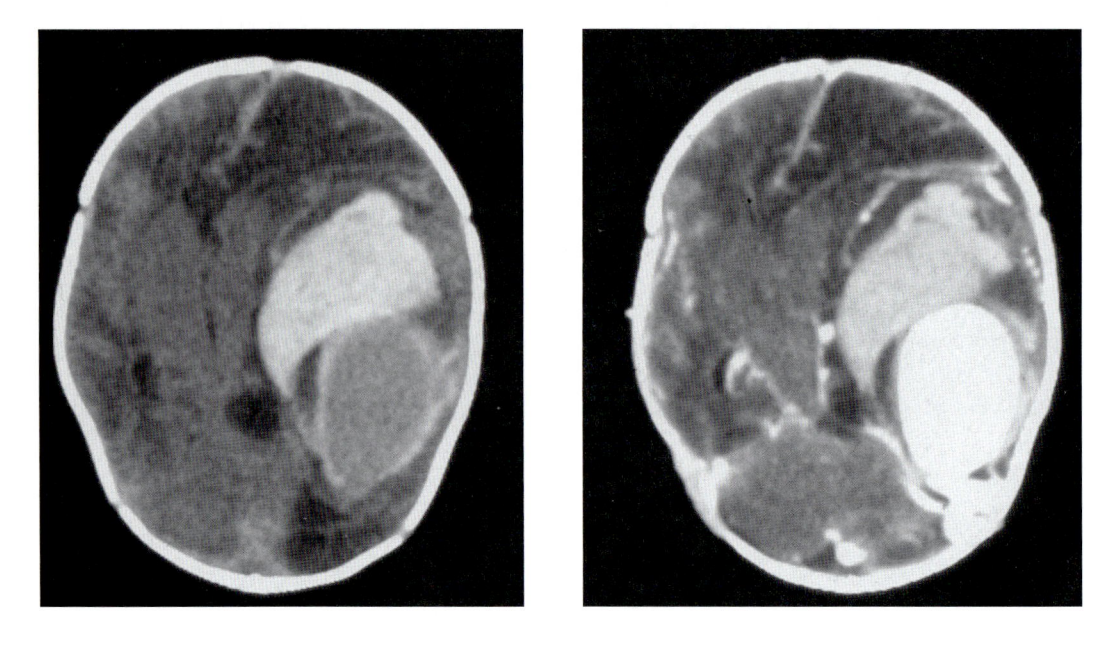

Figure 7.17   This male infant had a planned home delivery at 37 weeks' gestation with good Apgar scores, 9 and 10 at 1 and 5 min, respectively. However, the first hour after birth he was rather quiet. At 12 h of age he suddenly collapsed and needed resuscitation. On arrival at the hospital he was intubated and given phenobarbitone due to a suspected seizure. His pupils were noted to be asymmetrical.

(a) A cranial ultrasound examination (coronal views) was performed and showed a large parenchymal hemorrhage in the left temporal lobe, and a large echolucent area (asterisk) in the same region (3 cm in diameter). There was a marked shift of the midline with compression of the left ventricle. A Doppler signal was obtained in this echolucent area, suggesting an arteriovenous malformation.

(b) A CT scan confirmed the ultrasound findings showing enhancement of the arteriovenous malformation following administration of contrast. The lesion was considered inoperable and the child died. The father turned out to have a diagnosis of hereditary hemorrhagic telangiectasia (Osler–Weber–Rendu syndrome) and it is therefore likely that this child was also affected and had an arteriovenous malformation, a known complication of this disorder[150]

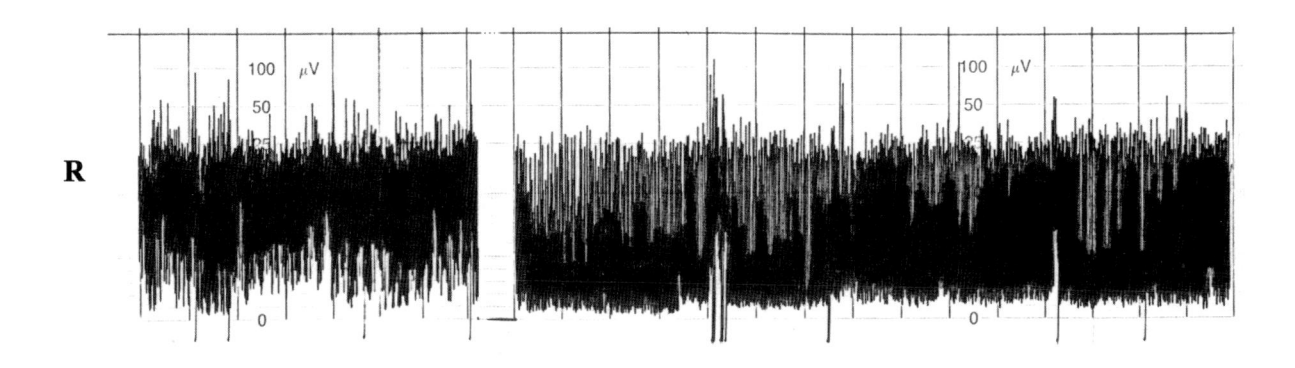

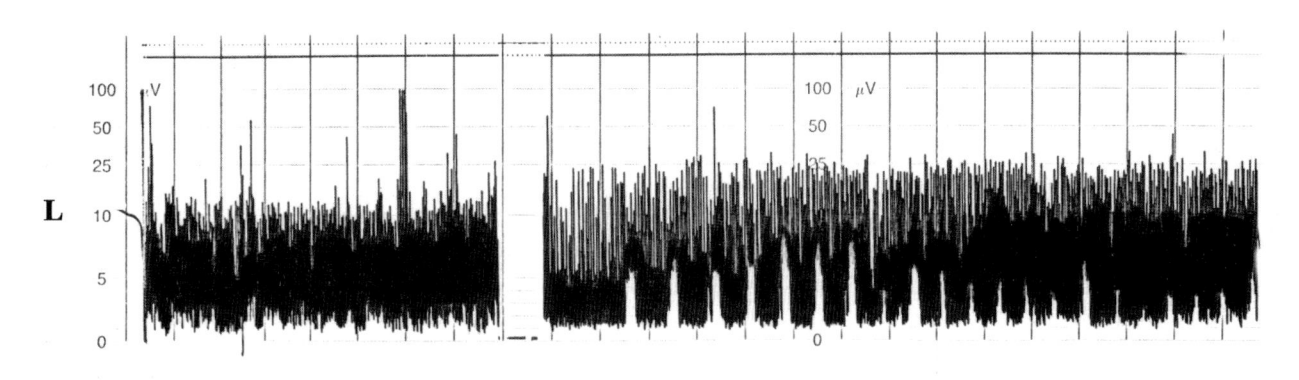

Figure 7.17 continued   (c) The aEEG was started, and due to the unilateral lesion, a bilateral recording was obtained from both hemispheres (R, right side; L, left side). The initial background pattern was mainly continuous although a clear difference can be seen between the two hemispheres with lower amplitudes on the left side (i.e. side of the lesion). Following the interruption in the recording, due to the CT scan, the background activity had deteriorated to a burst-suppression pattern on both sides. On the left side, repetitive epileptic seizure activity of 1–2-min duration at around 5-min intervals can be seen. On the right side there is no obvious seizure activity

Vein of Galen malformation

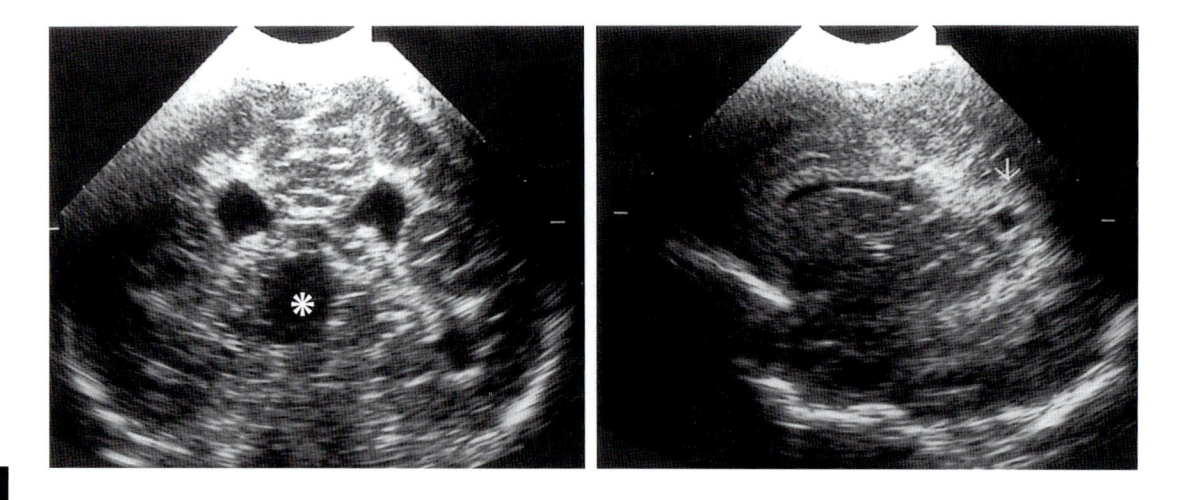

Figure 7.18 This female infant was born at 36 weeks' gestation. Her birth weight was 2640 g and her head circumference was 35 cm. Her start was good, with Apgar scores of 9 and 10 at 1 and 5 min, respectively. However, during the first few hours her condition gradually deteriorated. A chest X-ray showed severe cardiomegaly and a murmur was heard over the anterior fontanelle. She developed clinical seizures and received a loading dose of phenobarbitone. She was intubated and transferred to the NICU.

(a) On admission cranial ultrasonography was performed (coronal and parasagittal views) and showed a vein of Galen malformation (asterisk). Extensive ischemic changes were seen in the periventricular white matter. Localized cysts can also be seen (arrows). Because of the very poor neurological condition, this infant was not considered eligible for transarterial endovascular occlusive treatment and intensive care treatment was withdrawn

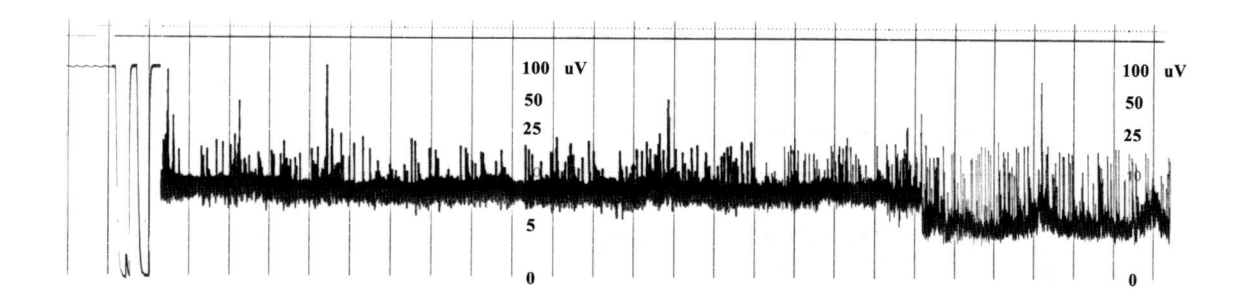

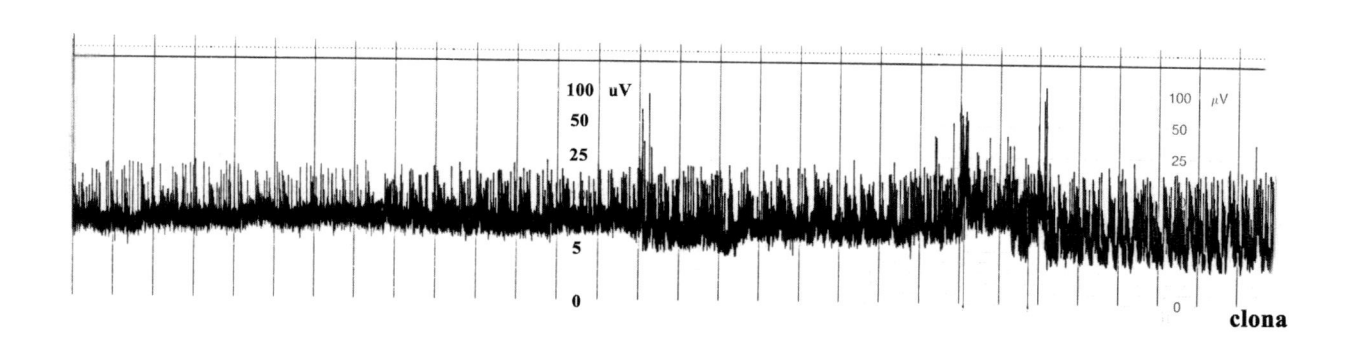

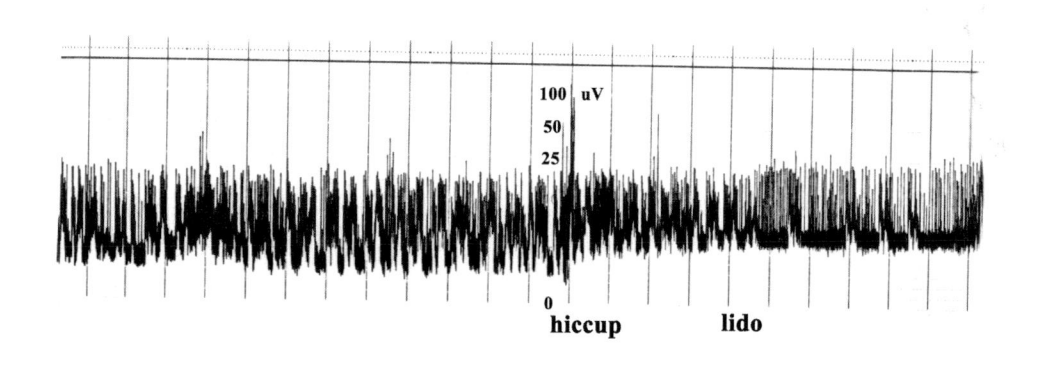

b

Figure 7.18 continued   (b) The aEEG was started when the infant was 8 h old after careful calibration, in order to have a correct baseline (see tracing). The initial background activity may, at first look, be misinterpreted as continuous with normal amplitude (between 7 and 10 μV). However, this is not a normal CNV pattern, but probably a low-voltage discontinuous burst-suppression pattern. It happens occasionally, in infants with very poor electrocortical activity, that the aEEG picks up extracerebral activity and adds up to 5 μV to the tracing, thereby lifting it from the zero line. If this is suspected, an EEG should be performed to verify this. This was not done in this case, but the continuing recording, which is severely abnormal, makes it very likely that the initial activity really was of very low amplitude. After 3 h of recording a more clear, but still quite low-amplitude, burst-suppression pattern is seen with the minimum level (probably incorrect) situated at 3–5 μV. On the second half of the middle tracing a seizure pattern emerges, with recurrent electrographic seizure activity but no clinical seizures. The seizure pattern was not affected by clonazepam (clona), but lidocaine (lido) reduced the seizure activity

Ohtahara syndrome

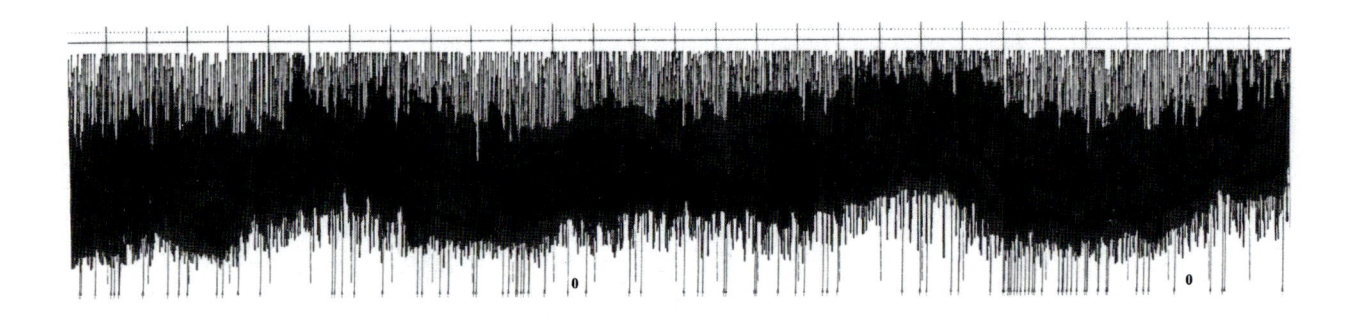

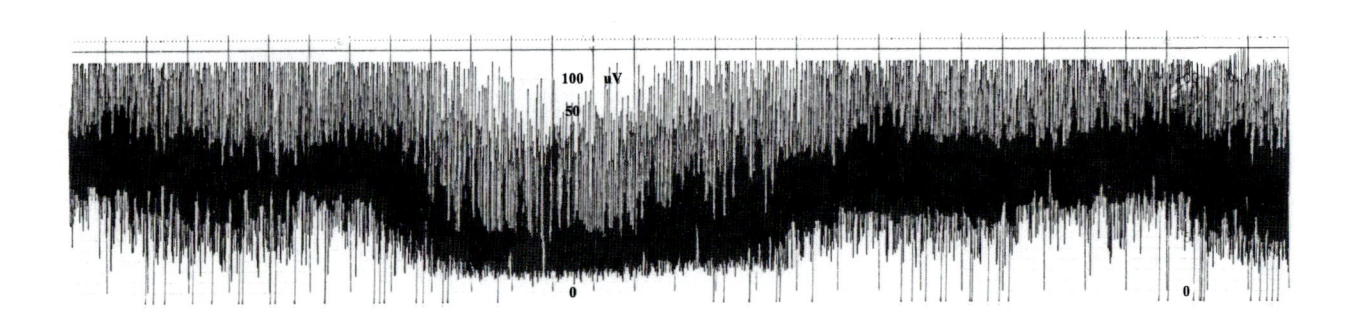

Figure 7.19 This female infant was born at 36 weeks' gestation following a pregnancy complicated by abnormal fetal movements and decreased fetal heart rate variability from 32 weeks' gestation. Her Apgar scores were 5 at 1 min, 7 at 5 min, and 8 at 10 min. Her birth weight was 2830 g. Her muscular tone was low and she developed seizures during the 2nd day of life. During her 2nd week of life she was transferred to the NICU for further diagnostic tests. Extensive metabolic investigations and neuroimaging studies, including MRI were carried out, but were all found to be normal. Several EEGs were done, showing a pattern compatible with Ohtahara syndrome.

The aEEG showed a severely abnormal background pattern for an infant of 38 weeks' post-conceptional age. The background was discontinuous with burst suppression of very high amplitude. Some variability can be seen but does not represent normal sleep–wake cycling

References

1. Steriade M, Gloor P, Llinás RR, Lopes da Silva FH, Mesulam MM. Report of IFCN Committee on basic mechanisms. Basic mechanisms of cerebral rhythmic activities. *Electroencephalogr Clin Neurophysiol* 1990;76:481–508

2. Maynard DE. EEG analysis using an analogue frequency analyser and a digital computer. *Electroencephalogr Clin Neurophysiol* 1967;23:487

3. Maynard D, Prior PF, Scott DF. Device for continuous monitoring of cerebral activity in resuscitated patients. *Br Med J* 1969;4:545–6

4. Prior PF. EEF monitoring and evoked potentials in brain ischaemia. *Br J Anaesth* 1985;57:63–81

5. Prior PF, Maynard DE. *Monitoring Cerebral Function. Long-term Recordings of Cerebral Electrical Activity and Evoked Potentials.* Amsterdam: Elsevier, 1986: 1–441

6. Agardh CD, Rosén I. Neurophysiological recovery after hypoglycemic coma in the rat: correlation with cerebral metabolism. *J Cereb Blood Flow Metab* 1983;3:78–85

7. Karnaze D S, Marshall LF, Bickford RG. EEG monitoring of clinical coma. The compressed spectral array. *Neurology* 1982;32:289–92

8. Aziz S, Wallace S, Murphy J, Sainsbury C, Gray O. Cotside EEG monitoring using computerized spectral analysis. *Arch Dis Child* 1986;61:242–6

9. HakeemVF, Wallace SJ. EEG monitoring of therapy for neonatal seizures. *Dev Med Child Neurol* 1990;32:858–64

10. Grundy BL, Heros RC, Tung AS, Doyle E. Intraoperative hypoxia detected by evoked potential monitoring. *Anesth Analg* 1981;60:437–90

11. Glaria AP, Murray A. Comparison of EEG monitoring techniques: an evaluation during cardiac surgery. *Electroencephalogr Clin Neurophysiol* 1985; 61:323–30

12. Murray A, Glaria AP, Pearson DT. Monitoring EEG frequency and amplitude during cardiac surgery. *Anaesthesia* 1986;41:173–7

13. Talwar D, Torres F. Continuous electrophysiologic monitoring of cerebral function in the pediatric intensive care unit. *Pediatr Neurol* 1988;4:137–47

14. Greisen G. Tape-recorded EEG and the cerebral function monitor: amplitude-integrated, time-compressed EEG. *J Perinat Med* 1994;22:541–6

15. Murdoch-Eaton D, Toet M, Livingston J, Smith I, Levene M. Evaluation of the Cerebro Trac 2500 for monitoring of cerebral function in the neonatal intensive care. *Neuropediatrics* 1994;25:122–8

16. Inder TE, Williams CE, Gunning M, Darlow BA, Gluckman PD. The relationship of electroencephalographic upper quartile cortical spectral edge frequency to the presence of white matter injury in the premature infant. *Pediatr Res* 2000;47:403A (abstr 2382)

17. Maynard DE, Jenkinson JL. The cerebral function analysing monitor. *Anaesthesia* 1984;39:678–90

18. Tasker RC, Boyd SG, Harden A, Matthew DJ. EEG monitoring of prolonged thiopentone administration for intractable seizures and status epilepticus in infants and young children. *Neuropediatrics* 1989;20:147–53

19. Murdoch-Eaton D, Darowski M, Livingston J. Cerebral function monitoring in paediatric intensive care: useful features for predicting outcome. *Dev Med Child Neurol* 2001;43:91–6

20. Wertheim DFP, Murdoch Eaton DG, Oozeer RC, *et al*. New system for cotside display and analysis of the preterm neonatal electroencephalogram. *Dev Med Child Neurol* 1991;33:1080–6

21. Reulen JP, Gavilanes AW, van Mierlo D, Blanco C, Spaans F, Vles JS. The Maastricht Cerebral Monitor (MCM) for the neonatal intensive care unit. *J Med Eng Technol* 1999;23:29–37

22. Jasper HH. The ten–twenty electrode system of the International Federation. *Electroencephalogr Clin Neurophysiol* 1958;10:371–3

23. Jasper HH. The ten–twenty electrode system of the International Federation. In *International Federation of Societies for Electroencephalography and Clinical Neurophysiology. Recommendations for the Practice of Clinical Electroencephalography*. Amsterdam: Elsevier, 1983:3–10

24. Monod N, Pajot N, Guidasci S. The neonatal EEG: statistical studies and prognostic value in full-term and pre-term babies. *Electroencephalogr Clin Neurophysiol* 1972;32:529–44

25. Westmoreland BF, Stockard JE. The EEG in infants and children: normal patterns. *Am J EEG Technol* 1977;17:187–206

26. Dreyfus-Brisac C. Neonatal electroencephalography. In Scarpelli EM, Cosmi V, eds. *Reviews of Perinatal Medicine*. New York: Raven Press, 1979:379–485

27. Torres F, Anderson C. The normal EEG of the human newborn. *J Clin Neurophysiol* 1985;2:89–103

28. Lombroso CT. Neonatal polygraphy in full-term and premature infants: a review of normal and abnormal findings. *J Clin Neurophysiol* 1985;2:105–55

29. Lamblin MD, Andre M, Challamel MJ, *et al*. Electroencephalography of the premature and term newborn. Maturational aspects and glossary. *Neurophysiol Clin* 1999;29:123–219

30. Selton D, Andre M, Hascoet JM. Normal EEG in very premature infants: reference criteria. *Clin Neurophysiol* 2000;111:2116–24

31. Hayakawa M, Okumura A, Hayakawa F, *et al*. Background electroencephalographic (EEG) activities of very preterm infants born at less than 27 weeks gestation: a study on the degree of continuity. *Arch Dis Child Fetal Neonatal Ed* 2001;84:F163–7

32. Connell JA, Oozeer R, Dubowitz V. Continuous 4-channel EEG monitoring: a guide to interpretation, with normal values, in preterm infants. *Neuropediatrics* 1987;18:138–45

33. Eyre JA, Nanei S, Wilkinson AR. Quantification of changes in normal neonatal EEGs with gestation from continuous five-day recordings. *Dev Med Child Neurol* 1988;30:599–607

34. van Sweden B, Koederink M, Windau G, *et al*. Long-term EEG monitoring in the early premature: developmental and chronobiological aspects. *Electroencephalogr Clin Neurophysiol* 1991;79:94–100

35. Ellison P, Franklin S, Brown P, Jones MG. The evolution of a simplified method for interpretation of EEG in the preterm neonate. *Acta Paediatr Scand* 1989;78:210–16

36. Viniker DA, Maynard DE, Scott DF. Cerebral function monitor studies in neonates. *Clin Electroencephalogr* 1984;15:185–92

37. Verma UL, Archbald F, Tejani N, Handwerker SM. Cerebral function monitor in the neonate. I. Normal patterns. *Dev Med Child Neurol* 1984;26:154–61

38. Thornberg E, Thiringer K. Normal patterns of cerebral function monitor traces in term and preterm neonates. *Acta Paediatr Scand* 1990;79:20–5

39. Hellström-Westas L, Rosén I, Svenningsen NW. Cerebral function monitoring in extremely small low birthweight (ESLBW) infants during the first week of life. *Neuropediatrics* 1991;22:27–32

40. Kuhle S, Klebermass K, Olischar M, *et al*. Sleep–wake cycling in preterm infants below 30 weeks of gestational age. Preliminary results of a prospective amplitude-integrated EEG study. *Wien Klin Wochenschr* 2001;113:219–23

41. Thiringer K, Connell J, Carter E, Levene M. Comparison between Medilog EEG and cerebral function monitor recordings on infants in neonatal intensive care. *Early Hum Develop* 1986;4:150 (abstr)

42. Hellström-Westas L. Comparison between tape-recorded and amplitude-integrated EEG monitoring in sick newborn infants. *Acta Paediatr* 1992;81:812–19

43. Klebermass K, Kuhle S, Kohlhauser-Vollmuth C, Pollak A, Weninger M. Evaluation of the cerebral function monitor as a tool for neurophysiological surveillance in neonatal intensive care patients. *Childs Nerv Syst* 2001;17:544–50

44. Toet MC, van der Meij W, de Vries LS, Uiterwaal CSPM, van Huffelen AC. Comparison between

simultaneously recorded amplitude integrated EEG (cerebral function monitor (CFM)) and standard EEG in neonates. *Pediatrics* 2002;109:772–9

45. Toet MC, Hellström-Westas L, Groenendaal F, Eken P, de Vries LS. Amplitude integrated EEG at 3 and 6 hours after birth in fullterm neonates with hypoxic ischaemic encephalopathy. *Arch Dis Child* 1999;81:F19–23

46. Thorngren-Jerneck K, Hellström-Westas L, Ohlsson T, *et al.* Cerebral glucose metabolism (CMRglc) and early EEG/aEEG in term newborn infants with hypoxic–ischemic encephalopathy. *Dev Neurosci* 2001;23:258 (abstr)

47. Bell AH, Greisen G, Pryds O. Comparison of the effects of phenobarbitone and morphine administration on EEG activity in preterm babies. *Acta Paediatr* 1993;82:35–9

48. Young GB, da Silva OP. Effects of morphine on the electroencephalograms of neonates: a prospective, observational study. *Clin Neurophysiol* 2000;111:1955–60

49. Hellström-Westas L, Bell AH, Skov L, Greisen G, Svenningsen NW. Cerebroelectrical depression following surfactant treatment in preterm neonates. *Pediatrics* 1992;89:643–7

50. Hellström-Westas L, Rosén I, Svenningsen NW. Cerebral complications detected by EEG-monitoring during neonatal intensive care. *Acta Paediatr Scand* 1990;Suppl 360:83–6

51. Benders MJ, Meinesz JH, van Bel F, van de Bor M. Changes in electrocortical brain activity during exchange transfusions in newborn infants. *Biol Neonat* 2000;78:17–21

52. Young GB, Campbell VC. EEG monitoring in the intensive care unit: pitfalls and caveats. *J Clin Neurophysiol* 1999;16:40–5

53. Groendaal F, de Vries LS. Selection of babies for intervention after birth asphyxia. *Semin Neonatol* 2000;5:17–32

54. Eriksson M, Zetterström R. Neonatal convulsions. Incidence and causes in the Stockholm area. *Acta Paediatr Scand* 1979;68:807–11

55. Legido A, Clancy RR, Berman PH. Neurologic outcome after electroencephalographic proven neonatal seizures. *Pediatrics* 1991;88:583–96

56. Hellström-Westas L, Blennow G, Lindroth M, Rosén I, Svenningsen NW. Low risk of seizure recurrence after early withdrawal of antiepileptic treatment in the neonatal period. *Arch Dis Child* 1995;72:F97–101

57. Scher MS, Aso K, Beggarly ME, Hamid MY, Steppe DA, Painter MJ. Electrographic seizures in preterm and full-term neonates: clinical correlates, associated brain lesions, and risk for neurologic sequelae. *Pediatrics* 1993;91:128–34

58. Connell JA, Oozeer R, de Vries L, Dubowitz LMS, Dubowitz V. Clinical and EEG response to anticonvulsants in neonatal seizures. *Arch Dis Child* 1989;64:459–64

59. Helmers SL, Constantinou JE, Newburger JW, *et al.* Perioperative electroencephalographic seizures in infants undergoing repair of complex congenital cardiac defects. *Electroencephalogr Clin Neurophysiol* 1997;102:27–36

60. Hahn JS, Vaucher Y, Bejar R, Coen RW. Electroencephalographic and neuroimaging findings in neonates undergoing extracorporeal membrane oxygenation. *Neuropediatrics* 1993;24:19–24

61. Connell J, Oozeer R, Regev R, de Vries LS, Dubowitz LMS, Dubowitz V. Continuous four-channel EEG monitoring in the evaluation of echodense ultrasound lesions and cystic leukomalacia. *Arch Dis Child* 1987;62:1019–24

62. Connell J, de Vries L, Oozeer R, Regev R, Dubowitz LMS, Dubowitz V. Predictive value of early continuous electroencephalogram monitoring in ventilated preterm infants with intraventricular hemorrhage. *Pediatric* 1988;82:337–43

63. Greisen G, Hellström-Westas L, Lou H, Rosén I, Svenningsen NW. EEG depression and germinal layer haemorrhage in the new-born. *Acta Paediatr Scand* 1987;76:519–25

64. Sheth RD, Hobbs GR, Mullett M. Neonatal seizures, onset and etiology by gestational age. *J Perinatol* 1999;19:40–3

65. Clancy RR, Legido A, Lewis D. Occult neonatal seizures. *Epilepsia* 1988;29:256–61

66. Volpe JJ. Neonatal seizures: current concepts and revised classification. *Pediatrics* 1989;84:422–8

67. Connell J, Oozeer R, de Vries L, Dubowitz LMS, Dubowitz V. Continuous EEG monitoring of neonatal seizures: diagnostic and prognostic considerations. *Arch Dis Child* 1989;64:452–8

68. Eyre JA, Oozeer RC, Wilkinson AR. Continuous electroencephalographic recording to detect seizures in paralysed newborns. *Br Med J* 1983;286:1017–18

69. Eyre JA, Oozeer R, Wilkinson AR. Diagnosis of neonatal seizure by continuous recording and rapid

analysis of the electroencephalogram. *Arch Dis Child* 1983;58:785–90

70. Hellström-Westas L, Rosén I, Svenningsen NW. Silent seizures in sick infants in early life. *Acta Paediatr Scand* 1985;74:741–8

71. Hellström-Westas L, Westgren U, Rosén I, Svenningsen NW. Lidocaine treatment of severe seizures in newborn infants. I. Clinical effects and cerebral electrical activity monitoring. *Acta Paediatr Scand* 1988;77:79–84

72. Mizrahi EM, Kellaway P. Characterization and classification of neonatal seizures. *Neurology* 1987;37: 1837–44

73. Volpe JJ. *Neurology of the Newborn*. 4th edn. Philadelphia: WB Saunders, 2001:188

74. Dennis J. Neonatal convulsions: aetiology, late neonatal status and long-term outcome. *Develop Med Child Neurol* 1978;20:143–58

75. Holden KR, Mellits ED, Freeman JM. Neonatal seizures. I. Correlation of prenatal and perinatal events. *Pediatrics* 1982;70:165–76

76. Clancy RR, Legido A. Postnatal epilepsy after EEG-confirmed neonatal seizures. *Epilepsia* 1991;32: 61–76

77. Ortibus EL, Sum JM, Hahn JS. Predictive value of EEG for outcome and epilepsy following neonatal seizures. *Electroencephalogr Clin Neurophysiol* 1996;98:175–85

78. Holmes G, Rowe J, Hafford J, Schmidt R, Testa M, Zimmerman A. Prognostic value of the electroencephalogram in neonatal asphyxia. *Electroencephalogr Clin Neurophysiol* 1982;53: 60–72

79. Finer NN, Robertson CM, Peters KL, Coward JH. Factors affecting outcome in hypoxic–ischemic encephalopathy in term infants. *Am J Dis Child* 1983;137:21–5

80. Rowe JC, Holmes GL, Hafford J, *et al.* Prognostic value of the electroencephalogram in term and preterm infants following neonatal seizures. *Electroencephalogr Clin Neurophysiol* 1985;60: 183–96

81. Holmes GL, Lombroso CT. Prognostic value of background patterns in the neonatal EEG. *J Clin Neurophysiol* 1990;10:323–52

82. Lombroso CT, Holmes GL. Value of the EEG in neonatal seizures. *J Epilepsy* 1993;6:39–70

83. McBride MC, Laroia N, Guillet R. Electrographic seizures in neonates correlate with poor neurodevelopmental outcome. *Neurology* 2000;55:506–13

84. Oliveira AJ, Nunes ML, Haertel LM, Reis FM, da Costa JC. Duration of rhythmic EEG patterns in neonates: new evidence for clinical and prognostic significance of brief rhythmic discharges. *Clin Neurophysiol* 2000;111:1646–53

85. Robertson C, Finer N. Term infants with hypoxic–ischemic encephalopathy: outcome at 3.5 years. *Dev Med Child Neurol* 1985;27:473–84

86. Wasterlain CG. Effects of neonatal status epilepticus on rat brain development. *Neurology* 1976;26: 975–86

87. Scher MS, Painter MJ. Controversies concerning neonatal seizures. *Pediatr Clin North Am* 1989;36: 281–310

88. Thoresen M, Hallstrom A, Whitelaw A, *et al.* Lactate and pyruvate changes in the cerebral gray and white matter during posthypoxic seizures in newborn pigs. *Pediatr Res* 1998;44:746–54

89. Holmes GL, Gairsa JL, Chevassus-Au-Louis N, Ben-Ari Y. Consequences of neonatal seizures in the rat: morphological and behavioral effects. *Ann Neurol* 1998;44:845–57

90. Huang L, Cilio MR, Silveira DC, *et al.* Long-term effects of neonatal seizures: a behavioral, electrophysiological, and histological study. *Brain Res Dev Brain Res* 1999;118:99–107

91. Wirrell EC, Armstrong EA, Osman LD, Yager JY. Prolonged seizures exacerbate perinatal hypoxic–ischemic brain damage. *Pediatr Res* 2001; 50:445–54

92. Shewmon DA. What is a neonatal seizure? Problems in definition and quantification for investigative and clinical purpose. *J Clin Neurophysiol* 1990;7:315–68

93. de Vries LS, Pierrat V, Eken P. The use of evoked potentials in the neonatal intensive care unit. *J Perinat Med* 1994;22:547–55

94. de Vries LS, Eken P, Beek E, Groendaal F, Meiners LC. The posterior fontanelle: a neglected acoustic window. *Neuropediatrics* 1996;27:101–4

95. Roberton NRC. Effect of acute hypoxia on blood pressure and electroencephalogram of newborn babies. *Arch Dis Child* 1969;44:719–25

96. Bunt JE, Gavilanes AW, Reulen JP, Blanco CE, Vles JS. The influence of acute hypoxemia and hypovolemic hypotension on neuronal brain activity

measured by the cerebral function monitor in newborn piglets. *Neuropediatrics* 1996;27:260–4

97. Watanabe K, Hayakawa F, Okumura A. Neonatal EEG: a powerful tool in the assessment of brain damage in preterm infants. *Brain Dev* 1999;21:361–72

98. Gavilanes AW, Vles JS, von Siebenthal K, *et al.* Electrocortical brain activity, cerebral haemodynamics and oxygenation during progressive hypotension in newborn piglets. *Clin Neurophysiol* 2001;112:52–9

99. Pressler RM, Boylan GB, Morton M, Binnie CD, Rennie JM. Early serial EEG in hypoxic ischaemic encephalopathy. *Clin Neurophysiol* 2001;112:31–7

100. Gunn AJ, Parer JT, Mallard CE, Williams CE, Gluckman PD. Cerebral histologic and electrocorticographic changes after asphyxia in fetal sheep. *Pediatr Res* 1992;31:486–91

101. Williams CE, Gunn AJ, Mallard C, Gluckman PD. Outcome after ischemia in the developing brain: an electroencephalographic and histological study. *Ann Neurol* 1992;31:14–21

102. Monod N, Dreyfus-Brisac C. Prognostic value of the EEG in fullterm newborns. *Handbook Electroencephalogr Clin Neurophysiol* 1972;15:89–100

103. Bjerre I, Hellström-Westas L, Rosén I, Svenningsen NW. Monitoring of cerebral function after severe birth asphyxia in infancy. *Arch Dis Child* 1983;58:997–1002

104. Archbald F, Verma, UL, Tejani NA, Handwerker SM. Cerebral function monitor in the neonate. II. Birth asphyxia. *Dev Med Child Neurol* 1984;26:162–8

105. Azzopardi D, Guarino I, Brayshaw C, *et al.* Prediction of neurological outcome after birth asphyxia from early continuous two-channel electroencephalography. *Early Hum Dev* 1999;55:113–23

106. Biagioni E, Mercuri E, Rutherford M, *et al.* Combined use of electroencephalogram and magnetic resonance imaging in full-term neonates with acute encephalopathy. *Pediatrics* 2001;107:461–8

107. Thornberg E, Ekström-Jodal B. Cerebral function monitoring: a method of predicting outcome in term neonates after severe perinatal asphyxia. *Acta Paediatr* 1994;83:596–601

108. Wertheim D, Mercuri E, Faundez JC, Rutherford M, Acolet D, Dubowitz L. Prognostic value of continuous electroencephalographic recording in full term infants with hypoxic ischaemic encephalopathy. *Arch Dis Child* 1995;71:F97–102

109. Eken P, Toet MC, Groenendaal F, de Vries LS. Predictive value of early neuroimaging, pulsed Doppler and neurophysiology in full term infants with hypoxic–ischaemic encephalopathy. *Arch Dis Child* 1995;73:F75–80

110. Hellström-Westas L, Rosén I, Svenningsen NW. Predictive value of early continuous amplitude integrated EEG recordings on outcome after severe birth asphyxia in full term infants. *Arch Dis Child* 1995;72:F34–8

111. al Naqeeb N, Edwards AD, Cowan FM, Azzopardi D. Assessment of neonatal encephalopathy by amplitude-integrated electroencephalography. *Pediatrics* 1999;103:1263–71

112. Thornberg E, Thiringer K, Hagberg H, Kjellmer I. Neuron specific enolase in asphyxiated newborns: association with encephalopathy and cerebral function monitor trace. *Arch Dis Child* 1995;72:F39–42

113. Shalak LF, Laptook AR, Velaphi SC, Perlman JM. The amplitude integrated EEG (aEEG) coupled with an early neurologic exam is an important adjunct method for enrollment of high risk term infants in neuroprotective strategies. *Pediatr Res* 2001;49:304A (abstr 1737)

114. Finer NN, Robertson CM, Richards RT, Pinnell LE, Peters KL. Hypoxic–ischemic encephalopathy in term neonates: perinatal factors and outcome. *J Pediatr* 1981;98:112–17

115. Biagioni E, Bartalena L, Biver P, Pieri R, Cioni G. Electroencephalographic dysmaturity in preterm infants: a prognostic tool in the early postnatal period. *Neuropediatrics* 1996;27:311–16

116. Marret S, Parain D, Ménard J-F, *et al.* Prognostic value of neonatal electroencephalography in premature newborns less than 33 weeks gestational age. *Electroencephalogr Clin Neurophysiol* 1997;102:178–85

117. Graziani LJ, Streletz LJ, Baumgart S, Cullen J, McKee LM. Predictive value of neonatal encephalograms before and during extracorporeal membrane oxygenation. *J Pediatr* 1994;125:969–75

118. Grigg-Damberger MM, Coker SB, Halsey CL, Anderson CL. Neonatal burst-suppression: its developmental significance. *Pediatr Neurol* 1989;5:84–92

119. Steriade M, Amzica F, Contreras D. Cortical and thalamic cellular correlates of electroencephalographic burst-suppression. *Electroencephalogr Clin Neurophysiol* 1994;90:1–16

120. Aso K, Scher MS, Barmada MA. Neonatal electroencephalography and neuropathology. *J Clin Neurophysiol* 1989;6:103–23

121. Aso K, Abdad-Barmada M, Scher MS. EEG and the neuropathology in premature neonates with intraventricular hemorrhage. *J Clin Neurophysiol* 1993;10:304–13

122. Sherman DL, Brambrink AM, Ichord RN, *et al.* Quantitative EEG during early recovery from hypoxic–ischemic injury in immature piglets: burst occurrence and duration. *Clin Electroencephalogr* 1999;30:175–83

123. Hellström-Westas L, Klette H, Thorngren-Jerneck K, Rosén I. Early prediction of outcome with aEEG in preterm infants with large intraventricular hemorrhages. *Neuropediatrics* 2001;32:319–24

124. Mercuri E, Rutherford M, Cowan F, *et al.* Early prognostic indicators of outcome in infants with neonatal cerebral infarction: a clinical, electroencephalogram, and magnetic resonance imaging study. *Pediatrics* 1999;103:39–46

125. Tharp BR, Scher MS, Clancy RR. Serial EEGs in normal and abnormal infants with birthweights less than 1200 grams – a prospective study with long term follow-up. *Neuropediatrics* 1989;20:64–72

126. Watanabe K, Hakamada S, Kuroyanagi M, Yamazaki T, Takeuchi T. Electroencephalographical study of intraventricular hemorrhage in the preterm infant. *Neuropediatrics* 1983;14:225–30

127. Clancy RR, Tharp BR, Enzman D. EEG in premature infants with intraventricular hemorrhage. *Neurology* 1984;34:583–90

128. Greisen G, Pryds O. Low CBF, discontinuous EEG activity, and periventricular brain injury in ill preterm neonates. *Brain Dev* 1989;11:164–8

129. Greisen G, Pryds O, Rosén I, Lou H. Poor reversibility of EEG abnormality in hypotensive preterm neonates. *Acta Paediatr Scand* 1988;77:785–90

130. Rutherford MA, Pennock JM, Counsell SJ, *et al.* Abnormal magnetic resonance signal in the internal capsule predicts poor neurodevelopmental outcome in infants with hypoxic–ischemic encephalopathy. *Pediatrics* 1998;102:323–8

131. Levene MI, Fenton AC, Evans DH, Archer LN, Shortland DB, Gibson NA. Severe birth asphyxia and abnormal cerebral blood-flow velocity. *Dev Med Child Neurol* 1989;31:427–34

132. Pierrat V, Eken P, de Vries LS. The predictive value of cranial ultrasound and of somatosensory evoked potentials after nerve stimulation for adverse neurological outcome in preterm infants. *Dev Med Child Neurol* 1997;39:398–403

133. Papile L, Burstein L, Burstein R, Koffler H. Incidence and evolution of subependymal and intraventricular hemorrhage: a study of infants with birthweights less than 1500 g. *J Pediatr* 1978;92:529–34

134. Rosén I. Ictal and interictal EEG in childhood epilepsies. In Sillanpää M, Johannessen SI, Blennow G, Dam M, eds. *Paediatric Epilepsy*. Wrightson Biomedical Publishing Ltd., 1990: 161–78

135. Tallroth G, Lindgren M, Stenberg G, Rosen I, Agardh CD. Neurophysiological changes during insulin-induced hypoglycaemia and in the recovery period following glucose infusion in type 1 (insulin-dependent) diabetes mellitus in normal man. *Diabetologia* 1990;33:319–23

136. Stenninger E, Eriksson E, Stigfur A, Schollin J, Aman J. Monitoring of early postnatal glucose homeostasis and cerebral function in newborn infants of diabetic mothers. A pilot study. *Early Hum Dev* 2001;62:23–32

137. Markand ON, Garg BP, Brandt IK. Non-ketotic hyperglycinemia: electroencephalographic and evoked potential abnormalities. *Neurology* 1982;32: 151–6

138. Holmqvist P, Polberger S. Neonatal non-ketotic hyperglycinemia (NKH). Diagnosis and management in two cases. *Neuropediatrics* 1985;16:191–3

139. Ohtsuka Y, Ohno S, Oka E. Electroclinical characteristics of hemimegalencephaly. *Pediatr Neurol* 1999;20:390–3

140. Yamatogi Y, Ohtahara S. Early-infantile epileptic encephalopathy with suppression-bursts, Ohtahara syndrome; its overview referring to our 16 cases. *Brain Dev* 2002;24:13–23

141. Baxter P. Epidemiology of pyridoxine dependent and pyridoxine responsive seizures in the UK. *Arch Dis Child* 1999;81:431–3

142. Hellström-Westas L, Blennow G, Rosén I. Amplitude-integrated encephalography in pyridoxine-responsive seizures. *Acta Paediatr* 2002; 91:977–80

143. Mikati MA, Trevathan E, Krishnamoorthy KS, Lombroso CT. Pyridoxine-dependent epilepsy: EEG investigations and long-term follow-up. *Electrocencephalogr Clin Neurophysiol* 1991;78: 215–21

144. Nabbout R, Soufflet C, Plouin P, Dulac O. Pyridoxine dependent epilepsy: a suggestive electroclinical pattern. *Arch Dis Child Fetal Neonatal Ed* 1999;81:F125–9

145. Mikati MA, Feraru E, Krishnamoorthy K, Lombroso CT. Neonatal herpes simples meningoencephalitis: EEG investigations and clinical correlates. *Neurology* 1990;40:1433–7

146. Eaton DG, Wertheim D, Oozeer R, Dubowitz LM, Dubowitz V. Reversible changes in cerebral activity associated with acidosis in preterm neonates. *Acta Paediatr* 1994;83:486–92

147. Hellström-Westas LK, Brun NC, Feet BÅ, *et al.* Effect of mixed acidosis on the EEG of newborn piglets. *Pediatr Res* 1996;40:533A

148. Klinger G, Chin CN, Otsubo H, Beyene J, Perlman M. Prognostic value of EEG in neonatal bacterial meningitis. *Pediatr Neurol* 2001;24:28–31

149. Ernst MR, Pekelharing M, Gooskens RHJM, Breslau-Siderius EJ, de Vries LS. Neonatale convulsies: niet altijd asfyxie. *Tijdschr Kindergeneeskd* 1997;65:259–64

150. Morgan T, McDonald J, Anderson C, *et al.* Intracranial hemorrhage in infants and children with hereditary hemorrhagic telangiectasia (Osler–Weber–Rendu syndrome). *Pediatrics* 2002; 109:1–12

Index